PRAISE
A BREAST CANCER JOURNEY

"A valuable, highly informative, and lucid compendium composed purposefully for fellow travelers."

KIRKUS REVIEWS

"*A Breast Cancer Journey* is a fantastic guide for anyone newly diagnosed with breast cancer. Packed with vital details for understanding a breast cancer diagnosis, planning treatment, and navigating recovery, Jennifer Douglas's book should be on every oncologist's shelf."

BEVERLEY ZAVALETA, MD
AUTHOR OF *BRAVING CHEMO: WHAT TO EXPECT, HOW TO PREPARE AND HOW TO GET THROUGH IT*

"Like having coffee with a loving older sister, Jennifer Douglas shares her experience, offers insights and advice, and provides a guided tour through the physical and emotional challenges of a breast cancer diagnosis, while never losing sight of the reality that cancer and the experiences it inflicts on us are as varied as we are. As you read, you can practically feel her comforting hand reaching across the table to give you a squeeze. A must-read for anyone with a diagnosis."

CYNTHIA HAYES
AUTHOR OF *THE BIG ORDEAL: UNDERSTANDING AND MANAGING THE PSYCHOLOGICAL TURMOIL OF CANCER*

"No matter how much support you get (or don't get) from family and friends, a breast cancer diagnosis brings with it overwhelming feelings of shock, fear, anger, and anxiety. Reading this book is like sitting down with a good friend who's been there. Its pages are filled with a wonderful blend of the author's personal experience and well-researched information to help guide your decision making, quotes from others who've also walked the walk, and practical tips and suggestions to make your experience seem a little less frightening and a little more doable. In a word, this book is about encouragement. As Douglas so succinctly writes: 'Cancer treatment is hard, even when the cancer is found early.' Truth—that's what that is. If you've been diagnosed with DCIS or early-stage breast cancer, you'll want this book on your nightstand!"

NANCY STORDAHL
BLOGGER AT *NANCY'S POINT* AND AUTHOR OF *EMERGING: STORIES FROM THE OTHER SIDE OF A CANCER DIAGNOSIS, LOSS, AND A PANDEMIC*

"You've been diagnosed with DCIS and are thinking, 'Now what?' Jennifer A. Douglas offers guidance, inspiration, and an invaluable resource for you. Follow Jennifer's breast cancer journey and make it part of *your* journey. This book is gem!"

LESLIE FERRIS YERGER
CEO AND FOUNDER OF MY DENSITY MATTERS AND AUTHOR OF *PROBABLY BENIGN*

"*A Breast Cancer Journey: Living It One Step at a Time* is a perfect book for a person who is newly diagnosed with breast cancer. It will become your best friend as you navigate your new breast cancer diagnosis.

It goes into detail on how to handle emotions as you are diagnosed, choosing a surgeon, when you should get a second opinion, learning about imaging, understanding what happens with a biopsy, diagnosis, surgical game plan what to expect on surgery day, post-surgical treatments, and how to navigate life after treatments are completed. I love that Jennifer talks about sex after cancer—one of the most important conversations that may or may not happen with your doctor. It is all about quality of life. This book will be an excellent guide and is easy to read."

DR. DEEPA HALAHARVI
BREAST CANCER SURGEON AND SURVIVOR

"This heartfelt and beautifully honest work documents the author's struggle with breast cancer from a stage zero diagnosis and the unexpected hardships, diagnostic trials, and difficulties she encountered. . . . One of the things I enjoyed most about the work was the narrative skill of the author, which makes it feel as though you're sitting down for a coffee with a wise friend who is willing to share her heart with you."

K.C. FINN
FOR READERS' FAVORITE (5 STARS)

"Jennifer A. Douglas writes a book to guide and answer most cancer patients' questions. She does so through her extensive research, personal experience, and inquisitive nature, which did not prevent her from asking questions concerning her diagnosis and treatments. . . . *A Breast Cancer Journey* is an informative book I recommend to those undergoing cancer treatments since it will equip you with essential tips and insights on living through the pain as you focus on complete recovery."

GRACE RUHARA
FOR READERS' FAVORITE (5 STARS)

a breast cancer journey

a breast cancer journey

LIVING IT ONE STEP AT A TIME

Jennifer A. Douglas

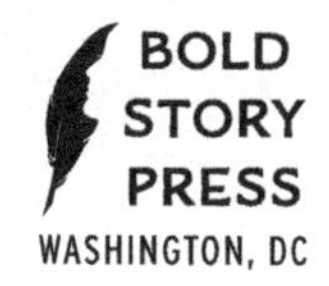

WASHINGTON, DC

Bold Story Press, Washington, DC 20016
www.boldstorypress.com

First edition: May 2023
Library of Congress Control Number: 2022920514

ISBN: 978-1-954805-40-8 (paperback)
ISBN: 978-1-954805-41-5 (ebook)

Text and cover design by KP Design
Author photo by Dan Douglas

Printed in the United States of America
10 9 8 7 6 5 4 3 2 1

To my husband, Dave,
and my sons, Ken and Dan.
Thank you for your love and support
every step along this journey.

To you, my reader.
I hope you find encouragement
and support in these pages
that will help you during
your breast cancer journey.

CONTENTS

AUTHOR'S NOTE

THE FIRST VERSIONS OF this manuscript had DCIS and stage zero in the title. But, as the book evolved out of a memoir of my journey and into what you hold in your hands today, the title changed to reflect the transformation. As I wrote this, I imagined having a one-on-one conversation with someone newly diagnosed with early-stage breast cancer. If you have been diagnosed with later stage, or metastatic breast cancer, your journey will look different from mine.

You will find descriptions of my treatments and appointments throughout this book. I have recreated dialogue in these scenes that reflect my memories of these events. I'll be sharing information about breast cancer along with these stories. I'm not a doctor, so please make sure to take all your medical questions to your care team.

Breast cancer is hard, no matter at what stage it is detected. I hope that you can find encouragement and hope within as you navigate the journey ahead of you.

INTRODUCTION

"LAST TIME THROUGH, THIS time with the lights!" announces my dance teacher with a smile. I twirl my hands above my head, move to the music, energized and enthusiastic. I hit the last pose with the instructors, my heart pounding, and my thighs twitching. Then, I tap "end workout" on my Apple Watch and slide to the floor of my bedroom. Instead of the applause I used to hear as a child after my performances, I hear my beagles snoring from their beds. I'm a year and a half out of an early-stage breast cancer diagnosis, and I can't believe that I'm dancing again.

The day before my forty-second birthday, I was diagnosed with ductal carcinoma in situ (DCIS). This type of breast cancer isn't invasive and hadn't spread to the surrounding tissues. It was a shock to be diagnosed with cancer. Instead of waking up on my birthday with a sense of hope for the future, I felt fear and anxiety. Would this be my final birthday?

What followed the diagnosis was months of imaging, biopsies, surgery, and radiation. After I finished with active cancer treatment in December of 2019, I had a renewed desire to build my stamina and increase the intensity level of my exercise. This was something constructive that I could do to rebuild my health after the destructiveness of surgery and radiation. These thirty minutes that I spend working out in my room have become a special part of my morning routine. Each time I do a dance or a high-intensity workout, I'm taking an active role in my recovery. And I have found the fun in exercising again.

I woke up on my forty-third birthday with hope. It had been a year since my diagnosis, and my active treatment had been completed nine months earlier. I remembered the moments of uncertainty, the nights of anxiety, and the worry, but they were not overshadowing my daily joy. I again had energy to dance and hope for the future.

If you had told me that I would be full of joy and energy after having cancer, I wouldn't have believed you. If you're just beginning your treatment, perhaps that idea is as far from your mind as it once was from mine.

WRITING THE BOOK I WANTED TO READ

I was overwhelmed when I first faced my diagnosis. I searched for books that would help me process this journey and help me feel less frightened.

I found some excellent books written by doctors that helped me understand the medical terms and treatment choices. These books helped me obtain the knowledge I needed to comprehend the breast cancer vocabulary. These reliable sources were well researched and offered me up-to-date information on the latest treatments available for breast cancer patients. Two books that were helpful references for me were *Dr. Susan Love's Breast Book* and *Breast Cancer: Real Questions, Real Answers* by Dr. David Chan.

But I also wanted to learn what it *felt* like to have breast cancer. I didn't have any close friends who had been through it, so I looked for memoirs on the subject. These books were written by women who had been there. They presented their stories with feeling and heart, and they also touched on the more intimate details of what it is like to have breast cancer. I particularly enjoyed *Better: How I Let Go of Control, Held On to Hope, and Found Joy in my Darkest Hour* by Amy Robach and *Bald is Better with Earrings: A Survivor's Guide to Getting Through Breast Cancer* by Andrea Hutton.

Both books were written by women who had been through extensive treatment journeys. I was in awe of their resilience and bravery, and grateful that my journey would likely be less harrowing. However, this didn't change the fact that I was terrified.

I longed for a book by someone who had been diagnosed with DCIS. My treatment team was positive and encouraging throughout the process, but I wanted and needed the first-person perspectives of women who'd been down this road before.

I decided to write a book specifically geared for DCIS and early-stage breast cancer patients. This is the book that I wish I had read during my treatment journey. I hope to demystify the treatment process, share resources, and offer insight into how I navigated the complex emotions and personal dynamics that arose during my treatment journey. Part One will explore diagnosis, treatment planning and surgery. In Part Two, I'll share how I'm navigating post-surgical choices and the ongoing challenges of recovery. At the end, I've included an appendix with my favorite resources for breast cancer information, supplies, and further reading.

If you scan the table of contents in this book, you will notice that I do not have specific chapters dedicated to chemotherapy or to metastatic breast cancer. My DCIS treatment experiences are woven into the fabric of this book. As I mulled over writing chapters dedicated to these important topics, I realized I couldn't share any personal insights with you. If you will be undergoing chemotherapy or are living with metastatic breast cancer, your treatments will be different than mine. In the appendix, I have included some selected resources on those subjects, including ones written by patients. I hope these will be helpful as you navigate your treatments.

The book follows my journey from where I was in my life at the time of my suspicious mammogram, through diagnosis, treatment planning, surgery, and recovery. In addition to sharing my experience and the treatment information I believe will be useful at each stage, I've listed my suggestions for optimizing your mental and emotional well-being relevant to that part of treatment. Throughout, I also share quotes from other people I've interviewed so you can get perspectives from lives that look different from mine.

Cancer treatment is hard, even when the cancer is found early. I hope this book can make it a tiny bit less so.

EXPECT TO FEEL OVERWHELMED

Facing a cancer diagnosis can feel overwhelming and scary. I was shocked at how many of my thoughts each day were filled with breast cancer. Before my surgery, I was able to have a conversation with Janna, another breast cancer patient. She had been diagnosed nearly four years before and was doing well. I distinctly remember what she said to me toward the end of our call: "Jennifer," she said, "you may not believe it now, but there will be days in the future where you won't be thinking about breast cancer all the time."

I laughed because I couldn't imagine a day like that.

As the time has passed from my active treatment, I have realized that my thoughts have cleared. I can look ahead to the future with hope. I'm able to laugh with my family again. Once again, I'm able to dance. Whatever brings you joy, I hope this book eases your journey in finding it.

PART I

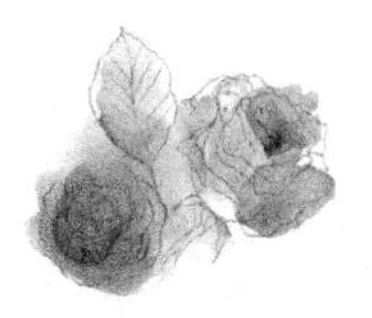

Diagnosis & Surgery

1

FIRST EMOTION
i'm overwhelmed

THE DAY AFTER MY breast cancer diagnosis, my husband and I were out to dinner for my birthday. I was turning forty-two, and we were sitting at our favorite restaurant to celebrate. Dave picked up his phone to snap a photo of me and share with a friend who had asked how I was doing. I smiled for the picture, and then, all of the sudden, the diagnosis hit me. I was overcome with fear and sadness. I wondered if this would be my last birthday dinner. Was I going to miss seeing my sons grow up?

I cried profusely. This wasn't just a few tears running down my cheeks. I was sobbing. My emotions were strong and raw. I think I cried right up until my steak arrived.

I had spent the previous day calling my friends and family, reassuring them that while I did have cancer, my prognosis was good. I didn't want them worrying too much. I felt like I needed to be strong and capable of handling this latest challenge. Whatever mask I had been wearing for those phone calls had melted away. In the intimacy of the dinner with Dave, I let it all out. I was terrified and overwhelmed.

FEELING OVERWHELMED? YOU'RE NOT ALONE

If you're feeling overwhelmed, terrified, angry, confused, or frustrated, you are not alone. As I have been getting to know other cancer patients, I have recognized a common thread of feeling overwhelmed. This emotion seems to be highest during the initial diagnosis and treatment-planning phases.

I quickly discovered that a Stage Zero breast cancer diagnosis didn't come with zero challenges. Along the way were challenging times. I discovered that I could lean on my husband, children, extended family, friends, neighbors, and church community in ways I had never done before. As my diagnosis became more public, I found out that there were cancer survivors all around me. These survivors came alongside me and offered me encouragement, listened to my struggles, and lifted me up in a way that I hadn't experienced before.

While I can't come to your home and have a cup of coffee with you, I hope that this book will encourage you as other women encouraged me. Each of us will have a unique diagnosis and treatment timeline. Here is how mine began.

MY JOURNEY: JULY 2019
THE ABNORMAL MAMMOGRAM

Summer was a good time for vacations and for taking care of my regular health screenings. Throughout the school year, I supervised virtual school at home for my two teenage sons, Ken and Dan. We began our virtual school journey when they were in kindergarten, and they were headed into ninth and eleventh grades in the fall of 2019.

I preferred to be home during the school day so I could be available for any questions they might have. It was easier to manage my medical appointments when school was out of session. I planned my second annual mammogram for the middle of the summer between our family vacation and a couples trip with my husband.

Our family had recently returned from a fantastic road trip through the Southwest. We had visited Arches National Park and ridden the Durango-Silverton steam train in Colorado. This was a family vacation that Dave had been looking forward to for years, and it had been a wonderful way to begin the summer. The memories of that trip were still fresh in my mind when I headed out to my annual mammogram in mid-July 2019.

I didn't expect anything abnormal, especially since my first mammogram had been uneventful. In my thirties, I had some fibroadenomas—benign lumps in my breasts that had been monitored. These felt like marbles and would roll around if I was doing a breast self-exam. They had been biopsied and weren't anything concerning.

I was happy that I was scheduling and attending my regular screenings. For years, I had been diligent about scheduling the visits for my kids but didn't bother with my own. I was comfortable putting their health as a top priority, but I didn't see the need to go to my own primary care doctor unless there was a problem.

I was surprised when that doctor called me the day after my mammogram. The radiologists had found something on the imaging and needed more information. After that call, I was a little anxious, but I figured that an ultrasound and a second mammogram would give them the information they needed to figure out what it was.

After the second round of imaging, which was a very uncomfortable diagnostic mammogram and an ultrasound, my phone rang again. It was my doctor, informing me that they were sending me to a surgeon. Everything sped up, and the urgency increased with each phone call. My first mammogram had been on Tuesday, the second on Thursday, and I headed to a surgeon on Monday. My anxiety rose as the appointments kept getting scheduled.

I had seen this surgeon a few years ago and didn't remember much about the previous biopsies except that I hated getting them. I wasn't convinced that I wanted to stick with this medical group because the surgeon I was referred to wasn't a breast surgeon. While I had my primary care doctor on the phone, I asked her if there were any other specialists in the area she might recommend. She was able to give me a few names to get started. I hung up the phone and made some phone calls.

Then I hit pause on the entire process. I didn't want to be recovering from a biopsy, or worse, get a cancer diagnosis while I was on vacation with Dave in the Caribbean. Our couples trip was coming up in just a few weeks, and while I could get in for the biopsy with the first surgeon before we departed, I wasn't sure I would be cleared to swim. In retrospect, this was one of the best decisions I could have made. It was a wonderful trip, and the last vacation we would take for more than a year.

DIAGNOSIS ISN'T ALWAYS A STRAIGHT PATH

From the very start, the diagnosis process can feel overwhelming and frightening. If you are feeling anxious, believe me, that is completely normal. Each procedure has the potential to change the treatment recommendations and inject unexpected problems and delays. This was worrisome to me at the beginning of my diagnosis process because everything was so new.

During the process, I discovered that there isn't always a straight line from imaging through biopsy and diagnosis to treatment. In my case, it was almost three months from my abnormal mammogram to surgery.

I discovered through my conversations with other patients that the treatment and diagnosis timeline can vary greatly from person to person. Things can move quickly, as they did after my initial abnormal mammogram or, if more imaging is needed, they can take months. Many breast cancer patients had their surgeries delayed during the initial months of the pandemic.

My diagnosis process took a while because I took a vacation before my first biopsy and changed medical teams. Initially, I was anxious about the delay, but in retrospect, it was a great decision. (I'll share more about why I changed teams in the next chapter.)

When I was feeling as if the process wasn't moving fast enough, I tried to go back to the image of a journey. This worked particularly well for me because, as I mentioned earlier, we had taken a long road trip in the Southwest before my abnormal mammogram. There were times when we ended up getting lost and took a little longer to get to the destination. I soon figured out that there were two ways I could handle the delay. I could get anxious, frustrated, and worried that I was going to be late. Or I could accept that we would get there when we got there. Eventually, I got to surgery and radiation, and those delays weren't significant enough to change my treatment. In fact, the delay made me more confident in my choices.

OTHERS' JOURNEYS
PATHS TO DIAGNOSIS

During my interview process, I had the opportunity to learn about other women's diagnosis process. It may be an abnormal mammogram that leads to a biopsy. Or perhaps a breast self-exam leads to a doctor's visit. The three quotes below are a sampling of the many stories I have heard from women when they share their diagnosis experiences.

jennifer f. "I believe my journey really began six months prior to diagnosis. I had just turned forty and made an appointment with my primary care doctor for an annual physical. I had some friends who recently turned forty as well, and they were having their first mammograms, so I figured I needed one, too. When I asked my doctor about it, she was a bit dismissive, explaining that given my age and lack of family history of breast cancer, I did not need to start regular screenings yet. That response did not settle well with me, and in retrospect, I wish I had followed my intuition.

"Fast-forward six months, and the world just started shutting down due to COVID-19. I was sitting on my sofa, braless, and reached down to put my shirt in between my breast and my chest because I was getting hot. I immediately felt what seemed like a marble under my skin. I was not checking my breasts regularly for lumps or bumps, but I was a bit shocked I hadn't noticed anything sooner because it seemed so large. I didn't think it was anything to be concerned with at first, but after about a week, I called and requested to be seen by a doctor."[1]

noelle "I had pain in my left breast and because I had recently stopped breastfeeding, I assumed it was pain from weaning off that process or a possible blocked milk duct. The pain was not constant, but if my baby boy crawled over or on me just right, the weight and pressure were unbearable.

"A couple of months later, I located a lump in a different area than where I was experiencing the pain; I could no longer ignore that something was not right. I went to see my OB-GYN for an exam."[2]

davita "I had just moved to California and started my new job in October 2019. My husband found the lump a little prior to moving, and I shrugged it off as nothing. I started working, and the lump started to hurt, so I had to find a doctor. I didn't know anyone, so I called my insurance company, and they helped me find one.

She ordered the mammogram, and then the radiologist ordered the ultrasound from there. From that point, they told me there was something alarming, and I needed more scans, an MRI, but the place they referred me to was booked for weeks. I went to one that was in my network, and they ran just about every test under the sun on me."[3]

Some of the common themes that run through these stories include fear, anxiety, and emotional distress. I remember feeling that my life stopped in the fall of 2019. I had many plans about what I was going to be doing, and cancer was not on my to-do list. Breast cancer was an uninvited intrusion on my calendar. As a result, I needed to let go of some of my commitments, ask for help in many areas of my life, rely on my family and friends in new ways, and focus on my physical, mental, and emotional well-being in intentional ways.

MENTAL WELL-BEING
MANAGING OUR NEW PRIORITIES

Throughout the book, you will find sections like this at the end of each chapter that specifically address mental and emotional well-being. Some of these are practical tips, and others are windows into my experiences. I hope that these can be helpful for you as you walk through the various phases of diagnosis and treatment.

One of the ways I addressed the feeling of being overwhelmed was to recognize that I had new priorities. My medical appointments took precedence over the other things in my life. I also needed to get organized. I discovered that if I wrote down the things in my head, I could calm down. I felt better when I focused on moving the diagnosis and treatment forward. Keeping track of my questions and to-dos in an organized way helped me feel less overwhelmed.

PRIORITIZE MEDICAL CARE & ACCEPT HELP

I was surprised by how many medical appointments I had as soon as the diagnosis process got going. I quickly learned that I needed to prioritize those appointments and accept help from friends and family.

My older son, Ken, was scheduled to take the PSAT during my diagnosis phase. I had three biopsies that week, two on Tuesday and one on Thursday. His PSAT took place Wednesday morning. There was no way I would be able to drive him to the testing location. I felt frustrated and angry. Cancer was taking away my ability to do "my job."

It turned out that I didn't need to let the frustration take over. My husband was happy to drive him to the test and pick him up in between his conference calls. My mom was in town, and she was able to take care of me after my biopsies.

I know Ken wasn't in the best of mental spaces during that test, and I felt like a terrible mom. I wanted to be there for him, which meant driving him to the site and being there to pick him up. That was so much of a part of who I was as a mom. But I was in recovery; I was in no shape to make that drive. When Ken came home from the test, he came upstairs to my room. He told me how he ran out of time on the math section and that there was someone next to him who napped through the entire test. I giggled with him as he told me the story.

This was the first of many times that I couldn't be a part of the boys' events in person. As time passed, I discovered that even though I couldn't be there, I could share in the emotional moments through their storytelling. I was able to enjoy their fun even while I was feeling lousy from treatment.

Prioritizing my medical appointments and accepting the help from family and friends were key steps in reducing my feeling of being overwhelmed. Accepting help wasn't always easy, but I look back in gratitude at the people who came alongside us during my cancer treatment.

MANAGE THE LOGISTICS

There will be appointments to schedule, phone calls to make, and research that you may want to do. You also might need to manage care for your children while you are going to appointments or recovering. Perhaps you need to schedule times off work. These are just some of the logistical aspects of being a cancer patient.

I ended up deciding on a time during the day when I would make phone calls and do scheduling. This helped me maintain my mental well-being. If I thought of something I needed to do, I wrote it down. Then I would take care of it during my next scheduled time to deal with logistics.

TRACK QUESTIONS & CONCERNS

I always seemed to think of the questions I wanted to ask my surgeon during my shower. That is not a very practical place to ask questions, so I would dry myself off and grab my phone to jot down the ideas. Another place that my questions surfaced was during my walks with Dave.

I needed a way to capture these questions and ideas so that I didn't forget them. I ended up using my phone to collect them. I could add to the list on my walk or right after I got out of the shower. Then I would either message my surgeon or ask him the questions during our next appointment.

As soon as I wrote the idea or question down, my mind was able to calm down and be less anxious. I was able to stop thinking about it and move on to something else. I discovered that writing down my worries, fears, questions, and concerns helped me improve my mental well-being. It enabled me to get them out of my head and move onto something more concrete.

ORGANIZE INFORMATION
CREATE A BREAST CANCER FILE

I recommend that you create a breast cancer file for organizing your paperwork, notes, and questions in one centralized place. I used a hanging file folder in my desk. It was right at the front of my files, so it was easy to access. When I had an appointment, I would grab the folder and place it into my designated appointment tote bag. My friend Judee gave me one that said "I'd Rather be in Paris" on it. I smiled every time I put that breast cancer folder into the bag, because it was so true. I would have much rather been in Paris!

It was helpful to have all my information with me during my appointments. Also, I was able to put the new papers into my folder right at the doctor's office. When I got home, I hung the file back in the drawer.

There's a lot that we need to keep track of during this cancer journey. If we develop systems that are easy to use, we can make it less of a mental strain for ourselves. These systems can reduce the feeling of being overwhelmed because we have a place to put all of the information.

EMOTIONAL WELL-BEING
RAW & UNFILTERED FEELINGS

I experienced raw and unfiltered emotions during my breast cancer journey, and you probably will, too. There were times I was peaceful and calm about it, and then there were moments when I was extremely frustrated and angry. I learned that it was almost impossible to fight these big, overwhelming emotions.

A few times when I was in the middle of a conversation with someone, I felt my emotional wall break down. I felt a wave of feelings come up as if I were about to explode. The person I was talking to had no idea what was coming.

I wish I could tell you that I walked away calmly every time. Or that I was able to tap into my inner peace and respond gently. That was not the case.

I had some emotional explosions during this time, especially during the diagnosis process. It was so hard for me to face the unknown. I was scared, and sometimes that fear came out as yelling and tears.

One of the things that helped me during the emotional times was staying in the moment. I would focus on where I was in the process. If my next step was a biopsy, then

I focused on preparing for that procedure. While I wanted to know how this breast cancer journey would end, if I dwelled on future procedures, I would feel myself getting panicked and frightened.

If you are feeling overwhelmed, you are not alone. After my abnormal mammogram and subsequent appointments, I, too, felt overwhelmed. In the next chapter, I'll share more about what it was like to change medical groups and seek a second opinion, and I'll introduce some of the medical providers you might see during your diagnosis and treatment. Once I had a trusted team in place, I felt my fear reduce.

2
CHOOSING A SURGEON & GETTING A SECOND OPINION

LESS THAN A WEEK after my first mammogram and follow-up imaging, I sat shivering in a paper gown in an exam room. My husband held the iPad, ready to take notes about the information we were going to get from this first surgical appointment. I had plenty of questions about my results.

The surgeon entered, greeted us, did an exam, and then agreed with the radiologist's recommendation for a biopsy. When I asked him follow-up questions about my report, he focused on reassuring me that it was unlikely that this finding was cancer but agreed with the radiologist that a biopsy was needed.

The appointment ended abruptly when the surgeon got called away for an emergency. As the door to the room closed, I felt my chest clench. I was uncomfortable with the way my situation was being handled. Something wasn't going right, and I needed to pause and advocate for the level of care I wanted.

MY JOURNEY
DECIDING TO ASK FOR A SECOND OPINION

Upon my return home from the first surgical appointment, I felt anxious and frustrated. I like to have time with my doctors to get my specific questions answered. In fact, I like to see specialists when I'm having a particular medical challenge.

I spent the rest of the afternoon trying to sort through my feelings. It wasn't until our evening dog walk that I found some clarity. I hadn't faced a potential cancer diagnosis before, but I had experience in delaying my own treatment to seek out another medical opinion.

Many years ago, I took a hard fall on some toys on Christmas Day. As soon as I landed on my right hand, I felt extreme pain. My first thought was, "I'm never going to play the flute again." Dave rushed me to the urgent care, leaving our two toddlers at his parents' house.

Unfortunately, I had broken a bone in my hand. When I mentioned that I was a musician to the doctors at the urgent care, they wouldn't cast me and instead urged me to see a hand doctor right away.

Finding a hand doctor who was working during the holiday season was a challenge, but after several calls, I was able to find one. He was able to look at the X-rays, tell me I was going to lose a millimeter of length in my middle finger, but that I didn't need surgery. After a cast and physical therapy, I was able to return to playing. My Christmas broken hand taught me the importance of finding a specialist.

LISTENING TO MY INSTINCTS

As I faced this new issue with my breast imaging, I realized that I was anxious because I wasn't seeing a *breast* surgeon.

I remembered the experience when I broke my hand and realized I wanted a specialist who would be able to sort out the benign and potentially malignant issues inside my breast. So, I made some calls and got an appointment scheduled. It took two weeks to see the doctor, but I was convinced that I needed to get a second opinion.

Although I didn't have any answers yet, I felt much more at peace. I felt like I had taken back some of the control I'd lost. By choosing to seek another opinion, I made a conscious decision to support my mental well-being even before a confirmed cancer diagnosis.

GETTING A SECOND OPINION: MEETING MY ONCOLOGIST & BREAST SURGEON

I met with the new doctor about my abnormal mammogram in early August 2019. This second opinion appointment was three weeks after my original mammogram. I didn't know what to expect, but I came in with my questions ready for the new doctor.

Dave was doing a lot of business travel during the late summer and fall, so my friend Rebekah came with me so that I would have another set of ears with me. She was a key part of my support team throughout my entire breast cancer journey. She came with me to appointments, drove me to biopsies, and brought mochas to cheer me up.

Rebekah and I sat down in the room, ready to meet the surgeon. Except he wasn't a surgeon; he was a medical oncologist. His specialty was working with patients who already had a confirmed cancer diagnosis. Now I felt silly! It turns out that I had made an appointment with the wrong provider. Do you recall in the previous chapter that

I mentioned being organized? Clearly, I didn't take my own advice. I felt foolish for making the appointment in the first place, and then I wondered if it would be a waste of time.

Thankfully, it was not. The oncologist looked at my imaging reports and took the time to review my most recent bloodwork. While he wasn't going to be the one to order a biopsy, he did notice some areas of concern in my chart that he wanted to follow up on. My white cell counts were low, and he wanted me to have some more bloodwork done.

Then he did a physical exam and talked about my imaging. He took plenty of time to listen to and answer my questions. He didn't rush me through the appointment. As the conversation continued, the knot of anxiety in my chest untangled.

I asked him if he would recommend a breast surgeon. His eyes lit up, and he said that he worked with one in this office. He had great confidence in this breast surgeon and would be happy to get me a referral. The oncologist walked out of the room, and then he popped right back in. The breast surgeon was in the office that day doing paperwork and would be able to see me right then. Was I willing to see him?

I was excited at this stroke of good luck. The breast surgeon came in, introduced himself, and then went right over to the computer to review my imaging results. I learned that this was his pattern in appointments. He would greet me and then get right on the computer to look over all the details. Once he was up to speed, he would move on to the next part of the appointment.

The surgeon performed a breast exam and then decided that the best thing to do would be to reorder all my imaging. I was surprised that he didn't want to just proceed with the biopsy. When I asked him why, he said that he always liked to make sure he had the most thorough and current imaging before making any other treatment recommendations. After I had my imaging redone, we would have another appointment to go over the results and take next steps.

His demeanor exuded a level of confidence and assurance that I hadn't experienced with my previous surgeon. Although I wasn't excited about redoing the imaging, I immediately felt that I could trust this breast surgeon, and I felt confident that this new team was going to be the right one for me. I left on vacation a few days later with the imaging appointments booked for the week I returned.

CHOOSING A MEDICAL TEAM FOR YOUR CANCER CARE

The breast surgeon is like the captain of the pre-surgery team. This doctor will be the one ordering the imaging and biopsies. But this will not be the *only* doctor who will be a part of your cancer care team. The breast surgeon will work in concert with other doctors who have different specialties.

Since I live in the United States, I am most familiar with how the medical system works here. Cancer referrals work differently in other countries. I will include a few resources in the appendix that may help if you live outside of the United States and are seeking care for breast cancer.

Cancer care centers are places where many different practitioners come together to provide the different aspects of cancer care such as imaging, chemotherapy, biopsies, and surgery. Many major metropolitan areas throughout the United States have comprehensive cancer centers that offer a patient the ability to have one centralized care team.[1]

If you are not located near a comprehensive cancer care center, or if it is not an option with your medical insurance, then I would recommend starting the process with the initial referral you get. Once you have identified your surgeon and are happy with that aspect of your care team, then the other providers can be found via referral.

Another important consideration when choosing care might be the location. An office that is located near your home or work can make the frequent appointments easier. Most of my appointments were at the office, which was close to my house. I was able to get to them quickly, and it was easier to arrange rides from my neighbors when I was undergoing radiation.

WHO MIGHT BE ON THE CANCER CARE TEAM?

There are several doctors and medical professionals who collaborate in cancer care, and it can be a little confusing when the referrals begin. Below is a general list of some of the care providers who might be on your medical team. You might see all of these doctors or only a few.[2] In addition to these practitioners, you should also keep seeing your primary care team because they will be important in helping you navigate any non-cancer-related medical questions you might have.

Surgeon. Responsible for ordering the imaging and biopsies. Works with the radiology team and others to determine the appropriate surgical plan. Performs the breast surgery and monitors your recovery. Breast cancer surgery can be performed by a general surgeon or a breast surgeon. All general surgeons are trained in breast surgery and may do additional training and fellowships in this area.[3]

Plastic Surgeon or Reconstructive Specialist. Responsible for the reconstruction part of the surgery. Will work with the breast surgeon and may be present during the initial surgery to perform the reconstruction after the cancer removal.

Medical or Clinical Oncologist. Specialist in diagnosing and treating cancer. Will work with the team to determine if chemotherapy is part of the plan. May order pathology and bloodwork. If you will be on endocrine therapy after surgery, this provider will order the medications and be the point of contact should you have any side effects.

Oncology Nurse. Specially trained nurse who guides patients through cancer treatment. This nurse may train the patient and family before treatment, be available during treatments to monitor vital signs, and be a point of contact should any questions arise about side effects.

Radiation Oncologist. Specialist in planning radiation treatment. Works alongside a team to design and implement an appropriate treatment schedule.

Radiation Therapist. Responsible for positioning the patient for treatment and administering the radiation plan designed by the radiation oncologist.

Radiologist. Interprets imaging, performs biopsies, and may perform the surgical localization process before a lumpectomy.

Radiology Tech. Takes the images for the radiology team. Might specialize in one particular type of imaging, such as mammography.

Pathologist. Interprets the tissue removed and evaluates whether it is cancer. Will identify biomarkers and other characteristics of the tissue that will be used to plan care.

Nurse Navigator. Works with the patient and the doctors to coordinate care. Acts as a point of contact for the patient when questions arise about treatment or scheduling.

Genetic Counselor. Helps patients understand the impact their genetics might have on their cancer. May order genetic testing and help the patient understand the results.

Primary Care Doctor. Coordinates with your cancer-care team as needed, performs any necessary pre-operative checkups, is a resource for any non-cancer questions you may have, and follows up with you during and after your treatment.

In later chapters, I will go into more detail about the doctors and techs I saw during my treatment. The most critical decision I made before undergoing my biopsies was to change surgeons. I am so thankful that I paused, reflected on my anxiety, and made a different choice.

A QUICK RECAP

To recap, these are some steps to make sure you are setting up a team you trust:

Research your surgeon. How many breast cancer surgeries does she perform per year? What types of reconstruction does she do? Is she in-network with your insurance?

Identify what is important to you in your patient-surgeon interactions. How easy is it to talk to the surgeon? Do you feel your questions are being answered? How responsive is your surgeon to messages or phone calls?

Pay attention to your emotions. If you are feeling rushed, disrespected, or dismissed during the appointments, don't ignore these emotions; they are signals that it may be time to make a change.

Before my cancer diagnosis, I had no idea that so many doctors, nurses, and medical professionals worked together to design and implement treatment. As you receive referrals for different aspects of treatment, I highly recommend that you check whether a provider or hospital is in-network with your insurance before undergoing treatment. This will help to minimize the out-of-pocket costs to you.

THE EXPENSE OF CANCER
FINANCIAL TOXICITY & TREATMENT

One important consideration to address before embarking too far into this diagnosis process is finances. Along the way, as I added new members to my team, I made sure that they were in-network with my insurance company. This reduced my out-of-pocket cost, which quickly added up.

Cancer treatment is extraordinarily expensive in the United States. According to an article on financial toxicity, "Cancer survivors usually report higher out-of-pocket spending than people who have not had cancer. Some cancer survivors report spending more than 20 percent of their annual income on medical care."[4] While screening for cancer may be covered with no co-pay, any additional diagnostic imaging, biopsies, or surgery will come with a high price tag.

Throughout my treatment, I had medical insurance through my husband's work. I had a PPO (Preferred Provider Organization) healthcare plan. Our family was responsible for 100 percent of the cost of care until our deductible was met, and then the plan would pay 90 percent of in-network expenses. Once we hit our out-of-pocket maximum, the insurance would pay all covered expenses at 100 percent.

I was shocked by how quickly we reached the out-of-pocket maximum on our medical insurance once my diagnosis began. In fact, one of the reasons I accelerated the move to radiation after surgery was that I didn't want to start over with a brand-new deductible and out-of-pocket maximum in January of 2020.

If you have medical insurance, I recommend that you look at your policy and understand what your coverage is. Will you have co-pays at each visit, or do you have a high-deductible plan that bills you after the services are done? If you do have a policy with a deductible and an out-of-pocket maximum, as I did, plan that your treatment will hit that out-of-pocket maximum sometime during this process.

If you aren't covered by medical insurance right now, I would recommend researching options to begin coverage before embarking on treatment. This might mean purchasing a healthcare plan on your own or looking into state-run programs, such as Medicaid. It can also be possible to negotiate cash prices with doctors and hospitals beforehand.

In addition to medical bills, unexpected expenses may come up during treatment that won't be reimbursed with medical insurance. Some of these may include parking fees, new bras, travel expenses, and extra household expenses.

I was thankful to proceed through cancer treatment while covered with medical insurance. That isn't the case for everyone. Sadly, medical bills are a leading cause of bankruptcy in the United States.[5] I'll include links in the resource guide to address the expense of cancer care.

Finding in-network doctors and hospitals can reduce your financial burden during cancer treatment. In my case, that meant driving to a hospital outside of Santa Clarita, California, where we lived, because our hospital wasn't in-network at the time. It added time to the surgery day but dramatically reduced our cost overall.

OTHERS' JOURNEYS
SECOND OR EVEN THIRD OPINIONS

I encourage you to take action and ask for second or third opinions, especially early in the diagnosis process. It can feel overwhelming to get thrown into cancer care, especially if this is new for you. Pausing and assembling a team that is right for you is time well spent at the beginning of this journey. Below are a few words of encouragement from other survivors:

sandy "I should've gotten a second opinion (about my reconstruction), but I was in a rush to get my surgeries scheduled before the end of the year due to insurance purposes. If you don't feel comfortable with your doctor, please get a second or even a third opinion. A good patient/doctor relationship is a must."[6]

noelle "My surgical oncologist was amazing! [He] made me feel supported every step of the way. My plastic surgeon was very dry and straightforward. I picked him because he is very well known and a professor for the campus. But this made seeing him post-op very difficult. I always saw one of his nurses. It was a breath of fresh air to see my surgical oncologist. My visits never made me feel like [I was] a number, and I was really listened to."[7]

jill "Never settle if you are uncomfortable with a doctor or treatment plan. You have every right to get a second opinion or a third for that matter. You deserve to find a team that works with you, includes you, and makes you feel like you are a part of your own care."[8]

lillian "Once I got my initial diagnosis, I was totally in shock. Since there were two lumps found in one breast, my surgeon wanted to do a mastectomy right away. At that point, I actually went to UCSF breast clinic for a second opinion, and the outcomes were similar. I didn't change my provider, but I'm glad I had a second opinion because it prepared me with some topics to discuss with my own doctors."[9]

davita "Do your own research and get a second opinion if you feel like you need one. This is YOUR life, and you are the one who has to live with your decisions, not the doctors. Take each day one step at a time."[10]

MENTAL WELL-BEING
PROCEED ONE STEP AT A TIME

I remember walking out of some of my appointments with a list of people to call, tests to schedule, and new information swirling in my head. Sometimes, I needed to sit in the waiting room or my car and take a few deep breaths.

If you are feeling overwhelmed, I recommend taking some time to write down what needs to be done. Then take the very next step and make one call to schedule that appointment. Another option would be to schedule the next follow-up appointment before you leave the office. That way, you already have it on your calendar and don't need to add another thing to your to-do list.

I found that proceeding one step at a time helped reduce the swirling anxiety in my head and helped me make progress in the right direction.

EMOTIONAL WELL-BEING
BE AWARE OF YOUR EMOTIONS

I discovered that my emotions before, during, and after my appointments and procedures were important to listen to. Once I changed surgeons, I realized that I would often feel relief after talking with him. My new surgeon took the time to answer my questions and was able to explain to me what the next steps were. This reduced my anxiety as I faced the unknown.

Negative emotions might be an indicator that it is time to seek another opinion. I encourage you to do that as early in the process as possible. It is much easier to seek a second or third opinion about treatment during the diagnosis process. I have spoken to women who have been told that a mastectomy is the only option, but then met with another surgeon who offered the option of a lumpectomy or a mastectomy.

Once you have met with your breast surgeon, there will be more planning steps along the way before surgery. This may mean more imaging and biopsies. Or, in some cases, it might be genetic testing or chemotherapy. In the next few chapters, I will address imaging, biopsies, genetic testing, and the other steps in the diagnosis process before surgery.

3

IMAGING
learning a new language (besides French) in my forties

I SAW THE IMAGING report pop up in my medical portal. Eager to discover what had caused the referrals for more testing, I read the following, "The new calcifications in the mid upper outer right breast are pleomorphic and amorphous and thus suspicious and need tissue diagnosis."

What was a calcification, and why did it matter that it was pleomorphic?[1] Searches online led me to complicated medical documents that I didn't fully understand. This was a new language, and I needed a way to understand what the radiologists were saying.

Breast imaging is a big part of the diagnosis process. A suspicious mammogram or ultrasound might lead us to even more screenings. I was surprised with how many different types of imaging were done during my diagnosis and treatment process. In this chapter, I'll discuss some of the different types of imaging that might be ordered for you and share with you the reporting scale that helped me better understand my imaging reports.

MY JOURNEY
IMAGING

I sat at my computer with several windows open on my large screen. On one side I had my mammogram report from 2018, and the other side I had the report from 2019. What was the same, and why did I need to go to a surgeon this year about these calcifications? I typed *pleomorphic amorphous calcifications* into the search bar and was pleased when some explanations showed up. I felt a surge of excitement through me. Maybe if I could figure out what they were I could avoid a biopsy.

Page after page led me to explanations that were incomprehensible. They were written in English, but they didn't give me any answers. I glanced at the bottom of the radiology report and noticed that the same radiologist had signed each of them. But there was no way for me to contact him. He wasn't available on my patient portal to take my questions. Frustrated, I closed the reports, and jotted my questions down in a notebook. There were no answers online that night.

I later had a doctor explain to me that the calcifications themselves were more like "cancer poop." They were indicators that something was going on in the tissue and needed more examination. If the report had said, "Looks like cancer poop," I would have better understood it.

As I have had more breast imaging since that July mammogram, I have learned a lot about what the imaging reports mean. I value reading the reports now that I better understand them. I still don't really know what *pleomorphic* means or why it is significant.

TYPES OF IMAGING

There are different types of imaging that can be ordered. If this is a regular checkup imaging appointment, then it will likely be called a **screening mammogram**. These are the mammograms that are regularly ordered once we hit the recommended age. They are done when there isn't a particular problem to look for. Screening mammograms are used to monitor changes in the breasts. In the United States, screening mammograms are typically covered under most insurance plans at no cost to the patient. As of this writing, the other imaging types may incur co-pays or co-insurance.

If there is a problem detected in the screening mammogram, then the radiologist will order additional imaging. This could be a **diagnostic mammogram**, which will get additional images of the area, an ultrasound, an MRI, or other scans such as thermography, PET, or CT.

No imaging is perfect, so radiologists may order a variety of imaging types to get the best idea of the abnormality. By the time I had finished my diagnosis process, I had many mammograms, ultrasounds, and an MRI. These additional imaging sessions came at a high out-of-pocket cost until I hit my insurance deductible for the year.

MAMMOGRAMS

In the United States, digital mammography has mostly replaced film mammography. This allows the radiologist to enhance, magnify, and manipulate the images. It also allows for these images to be stored digitally in your medical records.

Some radiology centers will offer 3D mammography. This is also called **tomosynthesis mammography**. It takes pictorial slices of the breast from different angles, and then reconstructs them using software to create the final image. Tomosynthesis mammography can find more cancers than digital mammography alone in breasts of all densities.[2]

Diagnostic mammograms use the same mammogram machine, but the technique is slightly different.[3] The radiologist has a particular area to focus in on. This may mean that the plates used to compress your breast are sized differently. Also, depending on the location of the abnormality, it may be more uncomfortable. The technologist may need to reposition your breast in different ways to get the compression just right.

I was really sore after my first diagnostic mammogram. The plates were positioned right up to my ribcage, and I felt that the pictures took longer. I needed to take pain relievers for a few days after the imaging until the soreness went away.

Sometimes with a diagnostic mammogram, you will have the ability to have a conversation with the radiologist about what she sees on the imaging. I found this extremely valuable. I was able to ask specific questions right after the imaging and leave the appointment with a clear understanding of what was going to be in the report that was sent to my surgeon.

If you are curious about how the imaging department handles the diagnostic appointments, I would recommend asking while you are making the appointment. I liked to know in advance if I would get the results right away by talking to the radiologist, or if I would need to wait.

ULTRASOUND

I have had a lot of breast ultrasounds! One of the longest ones that I had involved taking nearly fifty images. I was lying down on the table for a long time as the technologist got all the pictures she needed.

The **breast ultrasound** uses special sound waves to detect changes in the tissues. In a breast ultrasound, you'll be lying down on a table in a dimmed room. The technologist will place gel (which will hopefully be warm) on your breast and then use a wand to take the pictures.

The tech will take many photos and may adjust the contrast during the ultrasound. Once she is finished taking the photos, she will send them to the radiologist. Depending on the facility, you might have the opportunity to talk to the radiologist about your results.

In one of my ultrasounds, the radiologist came in and began doing the imaging himself. He wasn't sure what he was seeing on the still pictures, so he wanted to get more information.

As I had mentioned before, I had previous benign breast issues. These were identified and tracked using ultrasound. It can be difficult for mammograms to get a clear picture of breast tissues before a woman turns forty. Ultrasound allows the radiologists to get images even with the denser breasts many younger women have.

BREAST MRI

Despite its sensitivity, the **Breast MRI** is not standard practice in the United States before a cancer diagnosis. It is a time-consuming test and is also quite expensive. It does offer advantages over the mammogram and ultrasound, which is why it can be ordered after a cancer diagnosis.[4]

It is an excellent tool for detecting invasive cancer at an earlier stage. It can also detect changes in the lymph nodes near the breast. These changes can't definitively tell if the cancer has spread, but they can assist radiologists and surgeons with the planning. Breast MRIs can also see through dense breast tissue much better than a mammogram or an ultrasound.

However, false positives are quite common with a Breast MRI. There are abnormalities that can "light up" on the MRI. False positives may be reduced by timing the imaging in a very precise window of a woman's menstrual cycle. Ideally, the Breast MRI should be scheduled between days five and fifteen of the menstrual cycle.[5] This timing has been shown to reduce the false positives. This can be challenging because with a cancer diagnosis, there is added urgency in scheduling. I took the first available MRI appointment, and didn't pay attention to what time of the month it was. I wanted to get the appointment done so that my surgery could happen on schedule. In retrospect, it might have been better to wait a week and get it done during the right part of my cycle.

My surgeon ordered an MRI for me after my initial breast cancer diagnosis because he wanted to use it for surgical planning. Also, because I have dense breasts, he wanted to add in this imaging modality to see if there was any invasive cancer that hadn't been picked up by the mammograms or ultrasounds. Some surgeons order this test to verify if there is any cancer in the opposite breast before recommending a particular surgery.

WHAT IS IT LIKE TO GET A BREAST MRI?

I walked up to the check-in counter for my Breast MRI. "Could I see your insurance card and ID please?" the receptionist asked. Once I had pulled those out, she asked, "So, do you have any metal in your body such as staples, shrapnel, breast expanders?" I'm sure a bewildered look must have crossed my face.

"No, I don't," was what came out of my mouth. Inside, I was beginning to feel anxious. I had only had one MRI before, and it was not a pleasant experience because I felt claustrophobic. I was glad that my mom would be there to drive me home if I wasn't feeling well after the imaging session.

The tech called me back to the examination room and let my mom know that the wait would be about forty-five minutes. I was in for a long imaging session. He guided me to the dressing room and handed me a pile of MRI-safe clothing. "Please take everything off, including anything metal," he said. "There are two gowns and some non-slip socks for you to wear."

I asked if I could leave my underwear on. He said as long as they didn't have metal in them, I was able to leave them on. I checked my hair for any stray bobby pins, slipped on the grippy socks, and put on the oversized gowns. The first one I placed the opening in the front, and the second one I put on with the opening in the back. This MRI facility was co-ed, and the two gowns allowed me to preserve my dignity during the scans as I walked to the MRI room.

The humming of the machine greeted me as I walked into the scanning room. I looked at the setup of the table I would be lying on. It had a circular pillow and some blankets at the end of it. If the MRI tube hadn't been there, I could have been in a fancy spa waiting for a massage.

"You'll be lying face-down for the scan, with your breasts hanging through the table," the tech told me. "Before we begin, I'll need to place an IV for the contrast."

What? No one told me I would need to be poked for this scan. This was not in the brochure. I pass out with bloodwork on a regular basis, so I was not excited about the news.

"Um, okay, but I tend to pass out with blood tests," I managed to get out through my rising anxiety. I like to warn my techs before the fainting, so that they can be prepared. He had me sit on the table during the IV placement, and somehow I managed to stay conscious.

The IV is necessary because Breast MRIs are done with a gadolinium-based contrast agent, which is delivered via IV.[6] This contrast helps the radiologist interpret the imaging. There will be one set of MRI images taken without contrast, and then another set taken after they inject the contrast into your IV. I hadn't had a contrast-based MRI before, so this was a new procedure for me.

Once the IV was placed, it was time to get me set up for the scan. MRI machines are loud, so I was given foam earplugs to wear during the imaging. I had a hard time jamming them in my ears, so the tech helped me get them in place. I could tell they were working because it was hard for me to understand him while he was arranging me on the table.

Once he was finished helping me get in place, my head

was on the massage pillow, my breasts hanging loose below the table with an uncomfortable plate in the middle, my legs cozy under the blanket, and my arms loosely stretched out above my head. The tech had my right hand hold the panic button so that I could talk to him during the scan and had my left hand hold the IV tube.

"I feel like I should be getting a massage right now," I joked once I was in place. "Do you do spa services also as a part of this scanning?"

He didn't, but he offered me a nice warm blanket. At a few other of my MRIs, they offered me aromatherapy and asked what type of music I would like during the procedure. The soft scent of lavender transported me to an imaginary spa during the long scan.

Once I was positioned, the tech left the room, and then began talking me through the scans through the speaker. I was moved in and out of the MRI tube with the remote-control table. My role was to hold as still as possible. Before each one started, the tech told me how long it would take. Then the machine would begin making the rhythmic and loud clicking that indicated it was taking the images. There were several taken before the contrast was released into my IV. It felt a little cold in my arm when the contrast entered. Then the scans were all repeated.

I breathed a nice sigh of relief when the tech came on the speaker and told me that we were all done. He came back into the room and removed my IV. I was then cleared to head home. My results would be sent to my surgeon as soon as they were available.

The Breast MRI took about forty-five minutes from setup to finish. Depending on the facility, your scan may take between thirty and sixty minutes. I discovered that scheduling my Breast MRIs was challenging because I needed to take into consideration the time of the month and also find a facility with an open slot.

BREAST MRI RECAP

- Try to schedule between days five through fifteen of your menstrual cycle.
- Allocate about ninety minutes to two hours for the entire process.
- Ask for anti-anxiety medicine before the appointment, if you need it.
- Consider getting a ride to and from the scan.
- Leave valuable jewelry at home.
- Wear contacts instead of glasses, if possible.
- Prepare for the IV.
- Ask for comfort items such as a blanket, aromatherapy, music.
- Insert earplugs firmly in your ears.
- Get comfortable on the table before the scan begins.
- Remember that false positives are common.

TWISTS & TURNS: AN UNEXPECTED CALL FROM MY SURGEON

As more imaging is done, there may be a need for further imaging or biopsies. This doesn't always mean that the doctors have found more cancer. However, these discoveries can lead to delays in your surgery. That's what happened to me after my Breast MRI.

My mom and I were chatting as we put the bags from our shopping trip in the trunk. I had found some delightful rose hand lotion from France at a new store in the mall. It was a great day, especially since I didn't have any medical appointments on the book. I was about to start the car when the phone rang.

My heart sank when I saw that it was my surgeon. I had an appointment with him in two days. Why was he calling today?

"Jennifer, I just got the results back from your MRI, and they found some unusual things in the left breast (the one without cancer). Before we meet again, I'd like you to get an ultrasound on them. I've already put in the referral for you, so you can call and make that appointment."

I hung up the phone, shocked and frustrated. It was Tuesday, October 8. My surgery was on the calendar for October 16. There was no time to waste. I placed a call to the scheduling center. They were booked up at the Santa Clarita location but could get me in for imaging somewhere else in Los Angeles if I was willing to drive.

"Take the appointment," encouraged my mom. "I'll drive you." I decided to try another tactic before signing up for the hours-long drive. I called the imaging center directly and pleaded my case.

"Is there any way that you can squeeze me in?" I asked. "I'm happy to come anytime, and I could be there if you get a cancellation. This is urgent and might delay my surgery." Somehow, I managed to get those words out in a relatively calm tone of voice.

The scheduler wasn't able to make any commitments, but a few minutes later, my phone rang. "We can get you in tomorrow if you are willing to come in and wait," she said. "We can't give you a specific time, but if you're willing to come in at ten o'clock, we can squeeze you in. You may be in the waiting room a long time though."

"Thank you so much! I really appreciate it. I don't mind waiting!" I hung up, feeling victorious for getting something scheduled so quickly.

The next day, I got the ultrasound and was able to have a conversation with the radiologist afterward. Unfortunately, the results were inconclusive, and he was going to recommend additional biopsies.

On Thursday, I met with my surgeon. This was supposed to be my pre-op consultation. Instead, it was a debrief of my MRI results and a conversation about what was next.

I had three suspicious areas show up on my MRI, all in the opposite breast as the one with cancer. We had to delay my surgery, and I needed to have three more biopsies to determine whether those spots were cancerous.

According to the head of imaging in my medical group, my Breast MRI was one of the most complex she had ever seen. This is not a prize that I was looking to win. I love to be interesting, but not when it comes to medical imaging.

I was devastated that my surgery would be delayed. The only thing I could do was to get those extra biopsies done as quickly as I could so we could proceed with surgery with all the information needed. It took me time to walk through the emotions and then adjust my life again to accommodate for more procedures and appointments. Unplanned delays can happen at any time during our diagnosis, treatment, and recovery and are difficult to deal with. Over time, I've learned to make an initial plan and expect changes. When I approach my treatment with this more flexible mindset, I am more equipped to deal with the twists and turns that might occur along the way.

UNDERSTANDING YOUR IMAGING RESULTS

When I opened my first mammogram report and tried to read it, I was lost. It contained lots of words like "amorphous,""calcification," and "pleomorphic." I tried to figure out what the radiologist was describing by doing an internet search, but by the time I finished searching, I was more lost than when I started.

A DECODER KEY: THE BI-RADS IMAGING SCALE

Then, I discovered the BI-RADS imaging scale. This is an acronym for Breast Imaging Reporting and Data Systems.[7] The reporting scale isn't always included in patient-facing radiology reports because it was developed to communicate imaging results to ordering surgeons. However, with the new electronic health records, patients can now see these reports for themselves.

The BI-RADS imaging scale helped me understand my imaging results. I could estimate my cancer risk by looking at the number the radiologist assigned to each finding. This system was originally designed to be used only with mammograms but has also been expanded to include ultrasound and MRI reporting.

Because this scale is designed for communication between medical providers, your patient-facing report might not include the number. However, there are specific words in the patient-facing report that correlate to each number.[8] These are the words that I have included after the numbers. If you are still unsure about your BI-RADS score, please reach out to your ordering physician or radiologist.

BI-RADS SCALE, RECOMMENDATIONS & POTENTIAL PATIENT-FACING LANGUAGE

- 0 **Incomplete** Needs more imaging
- 1 **Negative** Continue with regular screenings
- 2 **Benign Findings** Continue with regular screenings
- 3 **Probably Benign** Recommended follow up in six months
- 4 **Suspicious Abnormality** May require a biopsy. Some radiologists may subcategorize this group into letter grades based on their suspicion as to whether the finding is malignant:
    - **4A** Low suspicion
    - **4B** Moderate suspicion
    - **4C** High suspicion
- 5 **Highly Suggestive of Cancer** Requires biopsy
- 6 **Known Biopsy** Proved malignancy

BREAST DENSITY

Breast density is an important consideration when interpreting imaging reports, because mammograms are not as sensitive and effective at picking up abnormalities in dense breast tissue. Individuals with dense breasts can have an increased risk of cancer.

Whether or not your breast density is included on your imaging report depends on where you live. Certain states and countries require this information to be included, and other places do not. There are four different types of breast tissue. I have included the approximate percentages of people with each type of tissue:[9]

A **Mostly Fatty Tissue** 10 percent
B **Scattered Dense and Fibrous Tissue** 40 percent
C **Heterogenously Dense** 40 percent
D **Extremely Dense** 10 percent

In general, the denser the breasts are, the harder it is for a mammogram to find a malignancy. If you read your imaging report and find out that you have dense breasts, it is important for you to discuss this with your doctor. There are other imaging techniques, such as a Breast MRI and ultrasound, that are better suited to find cancer in dense breasts.

I found that reading the reports wasn't enough for me to understand the purpose of all of the imaging. I made it a practice to ask a lot of questions about my results, both of the radiologist and of my surgeon. It helped me to better comprehend why additional imaging was being ordered. I also discovered that the communication was a good way to help maintain my mental well-being during the diagnosis process.

CHOOSING AN IMAGING LOCATION & RECEIVING RESULTS

Because the imaging will be used to help your surgeon make an effective surgical plan, I highly recommend that you get your imaging done at a location that can easily communicate your results with your surgeon. This could mean that the location will fax or electronically send the results to your surgical office. Or, if the imaging is done in the same facility, then the surgeon may be able to log in and see the results.

I decided to schedule my new mammogram and ultrasound at the radiology office that was in the same medical group as my surgeon. That way, he would be able to see the results as soon as they were available.

My surgeon liked to go over the results of my imaging and biopsies in person. He made sure that I scheduled follow-ups with him in the office a few days after each procedure. This gave us time to talk about results. On a few occasions, such as after my Breast MRI, he would call me if I needed to schedule further imaging before discussing the results.

If you would like to make an appointment to discuss results, please talk about this with your surgeon. Make a plan together, before anything is scheduled, so that you can know what to expect. Some options for communication of results include the following: appointment with your surgeon or radiologist, notes in the patient portal, phone call, or a letter.

OTHERS' JOURNEYS
IMAGING

While my imaging spanned the course of several months, that isn't always the case. Every woman I interviewed had a different imaging pathway that ultimately led to her diagnosis. Depending on the imaging location, you may proceed directly to more testing or a biopsy, or you might need to make an appointment for another day.

noelle Found a lump and had pain shortly after

weaning. "During my exam, my nurse practitioner did not notice anything abnormal and stated she just felt normal hormonal changes in my breast. Because I was also experiencing pain, the nurse practitioner wrote a referral for a mammogram, just for extra measure and precaution. Because this visit was so close to Christmas 2019, I put the mammogram on the back burner until after the holidays. Fast forward to March 13, 2020, and during a self-exam, I found a much larger lump in yet another area of my breast. At this point, I called my OB-GYN to ask if the referral was still good. It was, and they faxed it right over. I was scheduled for a mammogram and ultrasound on March 24. During my ultrasound, I was watching the screen, and because of my background working for breast cancer support programs, I immediately knew that the tech was measuring several locations on my left breast and left armpit. After my scan, she stepped out to have the doc review. The doc came in to see me and indicated that a biopsy was necessary due to possible abnormalities."[10]

jill "I had such bad anxiety waiting for my PCP office appointment that I ended up in the emergency room with chest pains a few days before Christmas of 2019; I told them my symptoms and they performed a chest X-ray, CT, and ultrasound while I was there. I had my mammogram the next morning. The following week I had a biopsy."[11]

lillian "When I went to my [imaging] appointment, I was immediately sent to [a] mammogram, ultrasound and biopsy. My insurance is Kaiser, so it's like a one-stop place."[12]

Our imaging pathways will all be unique, depending on where we are getting our care. Whether we are going straight from a mammogram to another type of imaging or need to get referrals along the way, it can feel like a lot to manage and can cause us to experience anxiety as we wait.

MENTAL WELL-BEING
APPOINTMENT LOGISTICS & COMMUNICATION

I went to the doctor often during my breast cancer journey. In fact, during my radiation treatment, I was going every day. There were a lot of logistics involved with appointments and communication. I developed a few techniques to help improve my mental well-being and help me feel less overwhelmed.

> **Pick your preferred appointment time and preferred location.** Because I was going to the doctor so much, I discovered that I had a preferred time for my appointments. I didn't want to go in the morning because that was the time that I set aside for coffee, dog walks, homemaking, and supervision of virtual schooling. I didn't want my appointments too late in the day because that risked running into cooking and dinnertime. I decided that 2 p.m. was the right time for my appointments. I was able to do my normal morning routine, eat lunch, drink coffee, and then get to my appointment. I would usually return home

in time to relax before dinner.

- You may not always be able to get your preferred time, but don't be afraid to ask. Unless you need to take the first available appointment because of a medical emergency, ask for the time you want. Sometimes, I will leave a message for my providers and let them know my preferred appointment time and date. If you don't want the 8 a.m. appointment, then ask for a different time!

- If you are in an urban area where there are different offices available, then think about which location is most convenient for your home and work. I spoke to one patient who chose her radiation location because it was midway between her work and her home. She would leave work, go to her radiation appointment, and then be halfway home already. This saved her a lot of travel time, which is important if you are fatigued!

Organize addresses and phone numbers. Make sure you put the phone numbers and addresses of your doctors in your phone contacts. That way, if the phone rings, your caller ID will tell you who is calling. Also, I would recommend having this information in the breast cancer file I mentioned in chapter 1. It is important to make sure your family or caregivers know where to find the information for your doctors.

They need to be able to find this information to help you get to your appointments and to contact the doctor in case of an emergency.

Sign up for the online portal. If your medical office has an online portal, I recommend signing up for it. The portal makes it easy to send a secure note to your doctor. There were times between appointments that I needed to contact my surgeon. He would read the note and then call me back. It was interesting to me that he preferred calling me, but it was an easy way for me to contact him with a quick question.

Plan your phone call time. There may be calls that you need to have with insurance or schedulers. Think about a time in your day when those calls will fit in. If you are working, it might be during your lunch break.

- I preferred to make these calls before lunch. This was a good time for me because I wasn't going to appointments in the morning. I would keep a list of who I needed to call and then take the time before lunch to get those done. I had a planned time to make phone calls, so I didn't need to spend mental cycles thinking about when I would get to that call.

- I discovered that having preferred times for calls and appointments helped me feel less anxious about everything I needed to do.

EMOTIONAL WELL-BEING
COPING WITH DIFFICULT EMOTIONS DURING THE IMAGING PROCESS

I dealt with unsettling emotions during the imaging process. I felt as if I were in a holding pattern above the airport. I knew a final plan would eventually be made, but the waiting was challenging.

FRUSTRATION

I felt frustrated during this time because I didn't have all of the answers. I would read and reread my imaging reports and still not be able to come up with a plan. I needed to come up with strategies to help me deal with the frustration before it turned into anger.

> **Phone a supportive friend.** I had a few people on my shortlist that I talked to when I felt emotional and frustrated. They listened to me without offering judgment or false hope. I recommend keeping a list of your support team somewhere convenient. When you are feeling frustrated or emotional and need someone to talk to, you can pull up this list and get some help
>
> **Do a physical task to work out pent-up energy.** It was helpful for me to do some physical work to get rid of nervous energy. Sometimes that meant picking weeds in my garden. Other times, I would clean

something dirty in my home. I was able to vent my frustration in the task and get something productive done at the same time.

Identify and deal with the source of frustration. Sometimes I didn't know why I was frustrated. Doing a physical task allowed my brain to wander so that I could begin to think about who or what was frustrating me. Then, once I had identified the source of my frustration, I would try to do something about it. Maybe I needed to talk to someone. Or perhaps I was frustrated because of the waiting and delays. In that case, there wasn't much I could do about it. It was helpful to know what was frustrating me, even if I couldn't do anything.

IMPATIENCE

There is a lot of waiting during the imaging process. We may need to wait for weeks to get into our appointments. Once the appointments are finished, we need to wait for the results. I felt a lot of impatience, especially before I had a solid surgical plan. These are a few techniques that helped me work through my impatience:

Embrace mindfulness. One of the things that I tried to do when I was feeling impatient was to be mindful of where I was in the moment. If I could slow down and focus on where I was and what I was doing, I could feel my impatience diminish.

Breathe for focus and calm. One simple way that

> I would slow my mind down when I was feeling impatient was to focus on my breathing. I would breathe in slowly for four counts, hold it for four, and then let it out for four. It took concentration to focus on my breathing, and that focus enabled me to calm down and be more patient. Sometimes, I would think about a Bible verse or an affirmation during my breathing that would direct my thoughts toward something calming.

I liked using these techniques when I felt myself getting impatient while waiting for appointments. Sometimes, I would be sitting in the imaging room by myself, without my phone available. I waited for the doctors to return to talk to me, but my things were put away on a chair or in a locker. I would first look around the room and really notice the surroundings. If there was artwork, I would take some time to gaze at it and notice the details. I would also pause and do some deep breathing. Mindfulness and deep breathing helped me to be more centered and focused once the doctor did arrive. Communication was easier when I felt calmer and less anxious.

Breast imaging is an important component throughout the breast cancer journey. I experienced a lot of imaging during the diagnosis and planning portion of my treatment. Now that I am post-surgery, it is a vital part of my monitoring process. My abnormal mammogram didn't result in an immediate cancer diagnosis. More information was needed, and that was gathered through my least favorite part of the entire process: core needle biopsies. In the next chapter, I'll share in detail about my experiences before, during, and after my biopsies. I'll also share what kinds of information the biopsies can reveal with the pathology reports.

4

BIOPSIES, SO MANY BIOPSIES

is this over yet?

AFTER IMAGING REVEALS AN area that is suspicious for cancer, the next step in the diagnosis process is usually a biopsy. A biopsy will remove a small amount of the area so that the pathology team can examine it and make a diagnosis. The first biopsy that I had in 2019 was by far the most eventful of the five that I would endure. This one was a mammogram-guided biopsy.

MY JOURNEY
BIOPSIES

Rebekah had picked me up early for this biopsy and dropped me off at the facility. I was grateful that the location was close to my home so that I wouldn't be gone too long. Dave was traveling for business, but I wouldn't be recovering alone. My sons and beagles would be home to support me.

I entered the biopsy room feeling anxious and unsure. The nurse showed me the chair that I was going to be sitting in for the biopsy. It was big and comfortable, and the mammogram machine was situated in the front. I was relieved that I wouldn't be standing up. The biopsy machine and the computers were to the left of the chair.

The radiology tech and the radiologist began getting me positioned for the biopsy. They placed my right breast in compression vertically, took some images to ensure the equipment was positioned correctly. I got curious and asked how the procedure would work.

"Well, we're going to take a mammogram, identify the calcification, then use the biopsy needle to extract a sample, then mammogram the sample . . ." Suddenly, my ears began to feel like they were filled with cotton and my vision got cloudy.

I had just enough time to tell the techs that I wasn't feeling well and then I blacked out. I sensed the medical team rush around me. One ran to get me juice, the radiologist held me up, and I felt the room swirling around me. I began to blink my eyes open as I was sipping on some orange juice. I asked them in a panic, "Did you get the sample?"

Thankfully, they did. Tears streamed down my face, and my body began to shake. I couldn't believe that I just passed out during my first biopsy. I still had one more scheduled that day. This was not the way I wanted to start the day.

I found later that vasovagal syncope, which is the medical term for passing out, is not uncommon, especially when a patient is sitting up for a procedure and is nervous. I felt anxious and talking about what was going to happen next didn't help. First, my heart rate and blood pressure dropped. Then, I fainted.[1] I learned that I should warn my medical team in advance that I had a tendency to pass out. That way they could prepare for my potential reaction. Thankfully, the rest of my biopsies were not as eventful, and I managed to stay conscious for them.

WHY ARE BIOPSIES NECESSARY?

Biopsies are a necessary part of the diagnosis process. They allow pathologists to obtain important information about an abnormality in the breast. I am glad that they allow for targeted and precise treatment. But I absolutely hated getting them. I despised being awake and aware of the process. I didn't enjoy getting the local anesthesia, and I found it challenging to manage my thoughts and emotions during the biopsies.

Before the development of the core needle biopsy technique, surgeons would use either a fine needle biopsy or a surgical biopsy. The fine needle biopsy doesn't remove as much tissue as a core needle biopsy, so it isn't as helpful with surgical planning. However, it can help a practitioner determine if a finding is a fluid-filled cyst. If more information is needed, then a surgical biopsy is ordered. A surgical biopsy needs additional planning and care because it is done under general anesthesia. It is a more invasive procedure and carries increased risk of infection.

The core needle biopsy technique was developed in the early 1980s and allowed for more tissue to be collected without the need for a surgical biopsy.[2] Pathologists are able to examine tissue samples and give initial staging reports to surgeons. Because these biopsies are done under local anesthetic, it is easier for the patient to prepare and recover.

There are other diagnostic techniques that are being researched, as well. There are certain blood tests, sometimes called liquid biopsies, that can detect tumor markers circulating in the bloodstream.[3] These types of tests are only helpful if your cancer is invasive. If you have a DCIS diagnosis (non-invasive) then there are no circulating tumor markers to test for. But, sometimes, an initial diagnosis of DCIS can lead to more testing. If your providers find invasive cancer on further imaging or biopsies, then blood tests might be ordered to check for tumor markers.

A biopsy is the only way that providers can tell if the finding in your breast is cancer or not. Generally, a biopsy will be ordered if your imaging has a BI-RADS 4 or higher.[4] These biopsies will provide your surgeon with preliminary pathological information on the tumor type, grade, hormone receptor status, and HER2 status. This information helps with treatment planning. I'll go more into details about pathology in the next chapter.

DIFFERENT TYPES OF CORE NEEDLE BREAST BIOPSIES

There are a few different types of core needle breast biopsies that can be performed to get a sample of the suspicious tissue. When a surgeon orders a biopsy, ask him which type you will be having. Each kind uses a different locating technique. In this section, I'll go over the commonalities between the biopsies, and then cover the differences.

GENERAL CORE NEEDLE BREAST BIOPSY PROCEDURE

These biopsies are done under local anesthesia. This means that you will be awake during this procedure, much like you are for many dental procedures. In fact, the numbing procedure is similar to that used in dental offices.

To minimize the bleeding during and after the procedure, you may be asked to stop taking certain medications for a week before the biopsy. Check with the ordering office to get accurate information.

The first step in the biopsy procedure is to check in and change into a gown. After that, you will be taken into the procedure room. This is a good time to let the medical team know if you are feeling anxious or if you have had an issue fainting during other medical procedures. This information will allow them to prepare for a potential event during your biopsy. Next, the technologists will do an imaging session. The purpose of this step is to make sure that the area to be biopsied matches up to the previous imaging.

After the area is located, the radiologist will sterilize the area and begin the numbing procedure. There will be an initial injection, called the "pinch and burn" shot. For me, this was the worst part of the numbing process. I really didn't like how the medication felt going into me. After the area is numb, there may be additional injections given to make sure that more of the tissue is numb. As this process is going on, make sure that you communicate with the doctors. If you are still feeling something after they have numbed you, please say something. It is acceptable to feel some pressure, but if you are noticing pain, let them know.

Once the numbing is complete, the radiologist will perform the biopsy. I'll address the specific procedures in each of the sections below.

After the final sample is taken, a marker will be placed inside your breast.[5] This marker is a very important part of the procedure. It notates the precise location of each biopsy taken. This marker can be used to aid a surgeon during a lumpectomy. It also can be viewed under a mammogram. Radiologists can see the marker and then reference your file to see which biopsy that finding is associated with. I have a few clips left inside me to mark my benign findings. Because there are clips on the specific findings, I don't need to have additional biopsies done. The only reason to order additional biopsies in a particular area would be if there are changes.

After the marker is placed, the biopsy needle will be removed. The radiologist will apply firm pressure to the area to stop the bleeding. The pressure might feel strange because you will still be numb.

Next, you will have some Steri-Strips placed over the biopsy area to close it up. After those are placed, you will likely have a mammogram. The purpose of this mammogram is to make sure that the clip is viewable. I didn't enjoy these post-biopsy mammograms. Once the radiologist confirms that the clip is in the correct location, it is time to get ready to go home.

At many of my biopsies, I was offered a cold pack to place inside my bra for the ride home. I got dressed and was ready to get home and get comfortable.

Now that I've described the general biopsy procedure, I'll go into the specifics of each different biopsy so that you can have an idea of what to expect.

MAMMOGRAM-GUIDED, OR STEREOTACTIC, BIOPSY

In this biopsy, a mammogram is used to locate the area to biopsy. It can be performed in two different positions: lying face down on a table with your breasts hanging below the table, or sitting up with the mammogram equipment in front of you. The office that did my mammogram-guided biopsy only had the option for me to sit in a chair.

The first step in the process is to get the breast that will be biopsied into compression. During a mammogram biopsy, the sample will be removed while your breast is compressed between specialized mammogram plates with holes in them. The opening allows the radiologist to insert the core needle into the correct area.

The radiologist and tech used a computer to make sure that the location was precisely calibrated. Once the area is numb, the biopsy tool is used to gather the sample. The sample can be imaged to make sure that it contains the right tissue sample. In my case, the goal of the biopsy was to remove some calcifications.

After the sample is removed, the clip will be inserted, and the compression will be released.

ULTRASOUND-GUIDED BIOPSY

If I had to choose a favorite flavor of biopsy, this would be it! I was the most comfortable during this one. During an ultrasound-guided biopsy, you will be lying down, usually on your back, on a table.

The tech will use the ultrasound wand to locate the area to be biopsied. Once she is clear about the location, she will bring in the radiologist. The radiologist will then confirm the area to be biopsied.

Depending on the size of the room, and which breast will be biopsied, the equipment might be draped over your body. I had one biopsy where there were four people in a room the size of a closet. The space was so tight that they placed some of the supplies on a sterile towel on my stomach. As the techs were passing wands over me and placing supplies on my belly, I felt more like an object than a person.

I found that closing my eyes during this biopsy helped me calm down, especially when the equipment was going over my body.

Once you are numbed, the radiologist will begin the biopsy procedure. This tool sounds like a staple gun. The radiologist will use the wand to locate the abnormality, then usually tell you there will be a loud clicking sound. You might feel pressure when the sample is taken, but you shouldn't feel any pain. Please let them know if it hurts.

The core needle biopsy tool can take multiple samples with one poke. You will hear a click each time a sample is taken. After all the samples are done, the clip will be placed, and the needle will be removed.

If a lymph node biopsy is ordered for you, the radiologist can use the ultrasound tool to locate a particular lymph node. I needed a lymph node biopsy on my left because the MRI picked up something. The radiologist used the ultrasound and chose one lymph node. When I asked her how she picked which one to locate, she said that she chose the one that looked the most suspicious. This sounded like more of an art than a science. But, since we have multiple lymph nodes in our breasts, it is preferable to sample the one that looks the most suspicious. Otherwise, we would be in for many more biopsies!

MRI-GUIDED BIOPSY

One of the abnormalities that showed up on my MRI was a finding that wasn't visible on either an ultrasound or a mammogram. This meant that the biopsy needed to be performed while I was in an MRI.

Of all the biopsies, this one was the most extensive and time-consuming. The first step in this process is to get you set up on the table, as if you were having another Breast MRI. The IV for contrast will be placed as well. The biggest difference with this set up and that of a standard Breast MRI is that your breast will be in compression, much like the mammogram-guided biopsy.

This compression is necessary to enable the radiologist to locate precisely the correct area to biopsy. Several MRI images will be taken to confirm the correct location. Then the radiologist will numb you.

The collection device sounds like a drill. The radiologist called it a whirring sound. I disagree. It really sounded like they were drilling out part of my breast.

Once the biopsy is finished, the clip will be placed and then you can get the placement mammogram.

If you had any challenges with anxiety or claustrophobia during a Breast MRI, please do not hesitate to ask for anti-anxiety medicine. This biopsy is quite time consuming, and it will be easier to handle if you are relaxed.

Once you are finished with your biopsies, you will get dressed and head home. I did appreciate that I was able to eat right after the biopsies. I often enjoyed a hearty meal to try to replenish my body. It was a great way for me to celebrate getting through these challenging procedures!

PREPARATION TIPS FOR BIOPSIES
PLANNING AHEAD FOR RECOVERY

During my weeks of biopsies, I discovered that I could recover more comfortably by planning ahead. Here are some of the things I recommend.

TRANSPORTATION

I suggest that you arrange for someone to drive you to and from your biopsy. Technically, you will be allowed to drive afterwards, but you will not know how you are doing until after the procedure.

For my first biopsy, I asked Rebekah if she would drive me and pick me up. She was able to do some errands while I was in the procedure because it took a few hours. I am so glad I did that because I was in no shape to drive after passing out.

DARK SHEETS

I woke up after my first biopsy and looked in horror at my bloody sheets. I had decided to sleep in a bra-style night-gown. That was a bad decision. Woozy, I got up from the bed and collapsed to the floor.

My bed looked terrible. My husband was away on business and couldn't help me clean up the mess. I needed help because I couldn't change the sheets due to my post-procedure restrictions. Embarassed, I asked my teenage sons for help.

Thankfully, they were good sports about it. "Mom, it looks like a crime scene in here," they exclaimed while pulling the linens off the bed.

After this terrible laundry incident, I went online and purchased dark colored sheets. If I was going to bleed again during my sleep, I didn't want to ruin my sheets! Trust me, invest in a set of dark sheets. You'll thank me later.

SPORTS BRA

I recommend that you have a few comfortable dark colored sports bras that you can wear after your biopsies. Front close sports bras will be easier to put on and take off after your procedure. I needed to be careful with big movements of my arm so that I didn't disturb the healing. If you don't have front close sports bras, you could step into your bra and pull it up. I wore a bra all day and night after my biopsies. This held my breasts in place and kept me from bleeding all over the bed again.

ACTIVITY RESTRICTIONS

I needed help with everyday tasks at home after my biopsies. I wasn't allowed to lift anything heavy or do lots of reaching. This meant that a few of my daily tasks were off my chore list. I wasn't able to do the following things:

- Laundry
- Dishes
- Cooking (I needed help getting the pots and pans out)
- Cleaning
- Gardening

- Changing sheets on the bed
- Walking the dogs

I was able to resume those chores about a week after my biopsies because the area had healed enough.

If you do not have help living with you, I would spend some time before your biopsy making some accommodations so that your recovery will be smoother. You might consider asking friends or neighbors if they can come in and help you out.

EASY MEALS

I was not up to cooking dinner after my biopsies. I either ordered delivery or had easy meals to prepare. This eliminated the stress of cooking and clean up. I also made sure that I had meals that were easy for my family to prepare on their own.

Also, if you have a friend, neighbor, or family member who is willing to make you a meal for your biopsy recovery, I highly recommend that you say yes! During three of my biopsies, my mom was visiting. She was a wonderful help in both the cooking and the cleaning. I was able to concentrate on recovery because she was willing to help.

COLD PACKS

I used cold packs on the day of my biopsy for the soreness. It helped to have a few of them in stock that I could rotate through. Your radiology office may send you home with some, as well.

HOME HELP

For the first couple of days after my biopsies, I was dizzy and exhausted. There were a few times when I had to stop and hold onto something so that I didn't fall down. I highly recommend that you have some help at home after your biopsies. Perhaps you could have a few friends give you a call or come and check on you during the first few days.

CARING FOR YOUNG CHILDREN

You won't be able to lift or carry your children for a while after the biopsy. Think ahead as to how you might want to plan for their care. This is especially relevant if you have babies who need diaper changes and baths. Another thing to think about as you head into your biopsies is how to plan for transportation for your kids to and from school and their activities. You might want to ask for help for a few days after your biopsy so that you're prepared.

SHOWERING

I wasn't able to shower for 24 hours. This was especially interesting on the week that I had three biopsies scheduled. I needed to make sure that I got a shower in on the day in between! I was really dizzy after, so I made sure that my husband was in earshot when I decided to shower. I didn't want to risk a fall while getting myself clean.

WORKING

I recommend planning for at least two days off of work to recover. The first day off would be your procedure day and then the second would be a recovery day. If you have a job that is physically demanding, then I would check with your ordering surgeon or radiologist to get specific recommendations for your situation.

Another option would be to schedule your biopsy for a Friday. You would have the weekend off to recover and likely be able to return to work on Monday.

After the biopsies, I was physically and emotionally exhausted. It was as if they drained my energy along with the sample. As I mentioned in the preparation tips before, I wasn't able to do many of my daily activities. I needed to ask and receive help from different sources.

SLOWING DOWN TO RECOVER

As I went through my weeks of biopsies, I realized that there was no use in fighting my fatigue. I had to accept that I was dizzy, weak, and exhausted. I also needed to actively participate in my recovery by resting.

I quickly found out that if I moved around too much or tried to lift things, I would hurt and bleed. On my first full recovery day, the one where I woke up to a bloodstained bed, I decided to try to walk around a bit and do a few activities. I overdid it. I looked at my biopsy site in the afternoon and realized it was bleeding more than I was comfortable with. It was a Friday afternoon, and I didn't know what to do.

I called the radiology office and asked them for help. They wanted me to come in so that they could look at me. Since my older son was home, I asked him if he could drive me there. I had no idea what I was in for, and I didn't want to pass out again and not be able to get home.

The radiologist saw me right away and offered to bind my breasts up with an elastic bandage. She told me sternly that

I needed to slow down. The more I moved around, the more I risked bleeding. Her strong words and my bloodstained bed were the encouragement I needed to stop trying to do so much.

Staying active was a coping mechanism. I was traumatized by my first biopsy, and I figured that if I kept my normal routines that I would feel better. I didn't want to appear weak, so I pushed through the fatigue. It turns out that I was making it worse. The best thing that I could do was rest.

PAIN MANAGEMENT

Ask your radiology office which medicines they will allow after the biopsy. Make sure you have those in stock and take them once you are done with the procedure. I carried the medicines in my tote bag and would take them once I got into the car. That way, when the local anesthetic wore off, I didn't feel as much pain. I ended up using acetaminophen for my pain relief because I was having multiple biopsies and that was the one I was allowed to take throughout the biopsy process.

I tried to stay ahead of the pain by taking the medicine at regular intervals. After about 24 hours, I would begin to taper the medication so that I could see if I still needed it. I also used cold packs after my procedure to help with swelling and to numb the area.

If you are experiencing extreme pain, please call the office for help.

APPROXIMATE RECOVERY TIME

During my diagnosis period, I had two waves of biopsies. The first occurred when I was diagnosed with DCIS, and the second wave was a week after my MRI. It ended up taking me about a week to feel fully recovered. The first few days were the most challenging. I had some biopsies that were sore for longer than others. But recovery varies greatly from person to person. It might take you a different amount of time to recover.

Once I learned my lesson about doing too much the first day, I changed my recovery tactics. On the day of the biopsy, I would come home and go straight to the bed or the couch. I would get up every hour or so to walk around, but other than that, it was a rest day. I also made sure to wrap my breasts before bed so that they didn't shift around at night.

I added slow walking back into my routine on the day after the biopsy, but I didn't walk the dogs myself, and I made sure that I wasn't having balance issues. The walking was nice to get me up and out of the house, and I was able to gauge my physical recovery with my stamina on the walks.

OTHERS' JOURNEYS
BIOPSIES & RESULTS

Waiting for results is extremely difficult. We are balancing the recovery from the procedure with our anxieties about what the pathology might be. Sometimes even the medical teams aren't sure how to communicate results to us. It can help to practice self-care and self-advocacy as we walk through the time between biopsy and results.

davita "Then I [had] my biopsy, there at the scan place. They flew in a doctor who specialized in breast biopsies. On November 20, 2019, I got the call. She wasn't my doctor, so she told me to find a breast surgeon and plastic surgeon stat."[6]

noelle "The next day [after my imaging], I had three areas biopsied (two in my breast and one in my underarm). Talk about pain! Waiting for results was hell as it was done on a Friday and [I] had all weekend to worry about it. When I didn't receive a call by noon on Monday, I called the Nurse Navigator at the imaging center for answers. The call went to voicemail every time I called. My husband also called as he was worried for me. Apparently, the Nurse Navigator thought my OB-GYN Nurse Practitioner was going to call me with the results and vice versa. At 4:58pm, my OB-GYN NP called to make sure I got the results. I told her I had not, and she then said the words I was dreading 'Unfortunately, this is cancer.'"[7]

sue Had first diagnosis with breast cancer in 1998 and another in October 2020. "Since 1998, my first diagnosis, I have had 6 biopsies. Each time, I held my breath for the results which turned out to be negative. In October of 2020, it was positive. I took a really deep fall into deep depression. I went down so many rabbit holes during treatments. What I learned is to:

1. Ask for help.
2. Self-care first.
3. Talking to a therapist is good.
4. Stop blaming myself; It's not my fault.
5. Meditation is a reset for my brain."[8]

MENTAL WELL-BEING
WAITING FOR RESULTS & PLANNING AHEAD

I had a really hard time waiting for results. I wanted to know right away what they were, but sometimes between a few days to a week was required to get pathology results. One of the things I did was to plan ahead with my surgeon and radiologist to make sure that I would get the results communicated to me in a way I was comfortable with.

RESULTS MANAGEMENT

I did not want to learn that I had cancer over the phone. I also didn't want to read that I had cancer on my online portal. So, I took active steps to make sure that this didn't happen. I made an appointment with my surgeon for several days after my biopsy to discuss results. If I called the office to see if my results were *in*, I specifically told the nurse that I didn't want to know what the results *were*. They respected my wishes, and I was able to find out *in person* that I had cancer.

In April 2021, the 21st Century Cures Act OpenNotes legislation went into effect in the United States that allows patients open access to all of their healthcare notes, including lab and pathology narratives. This means that you will have access to these reports on your online portal with the notes from your doctors. It is up to you to decide if you'd like to read these notes before your appointment or if you'd like to wait and discuss them in person.[9]

I decided not to check the online patient portal. This took mental discipline, but it was well worth it. My diagnosis took place before the legislation went into effect, so my results weren't automatically reported.

I was able to focus on recovery and not worry about when I would find out. I was still pretty anxious, but I wasn't looking at my phone every three minutes waiting for a phone call.

PLANNING AHEAD

Another thing that I did in between the biopsy and the results appointment was to research what kind of results I might have. I used the time while I was waiting to learn what kinds of cancer there were and what the biopsy might reveal. I will include some resources in the appendix that I found useful when doing my own research. Doing this research was helpful because I was familiar with the medical terms when I went into the appointment with the surgeon. In the next chapter, I will explain some of those terms so that you'll have more information going into that appointment with your surgeon.

EMOTIONAL WELL-BEING

RECOGNIZING FEAR, ANXIETY & WORRY

During the biopsy phase, I felt fear, anxiety, and worry. I discovered that I would have a physical response to these strong emotions. I could feel my chest constrict when my emotions heightened. I used some strategies during and after the biopsies to help me manage my fears.

CONNECT WITH THE MEDICAL TEAM

One of the things that I tried to do was to connect on an emotional level with my medical team. My friend Claire, who had been through cancer before me, encouraged me to make friends with all of the nurses. I took that advice to heart. I didn't always feel my best when I saw the team, but I tried to connect with each of my caregivers as much as possible. I would make small talk with them as they walked me back to the procedure rooms.

There weren't any friends or family going into the biopsy rooms with me. It was just me and the medical team. I tried to make conversation with the teams to get to know them and talk about how I was doing. This helped me feel less anxiety throughout the biopsies. I found that they were willing to come alongside and be supportive of me because I was vulnerable with them. I also made sure they knew that I might pass out. Many of them were understanding of my challenges and made sure to position me safely for IV placement and blood draws.

MEDITATE

Before my breast cancer diagnosis, I was not a meditator. I had read plenty of articles that described the mental health benefits of meditating.[10] But I hadn't felt the need to take the time for it. Also, I wasn't sure how meditation would be different from praying, which I did regularly.

As I became more familiar with meditation, I found that it was a way for me to listen and get in touch with my thoughts and physical sensations. In contrast, prayer was a way for me to actively talk to God and express my feelings. I found that meditation and prayer were both excellent tools to help me return to a state of calm.

Because I was getting emotional and anxious during my diagnosis period, I decided to give meditation a try. I found some apps on my phone that had guided meditations I could listen to. I'll include some of my favorites in the appendix. It took a little trial and error to find ones that were beneficial.

What I liked about the guided meditations was the imagery that they would give during the sessions. I had difficulty falling asleep, and I tried a relaxing meditation one night. It guided me to envision a windmill in a field and then let the windmill blow my worries away. I listened to it a few times, but after that I was able to bring up the image in my mind on my own. I really liked having an image in my mind that I could use to help me let go of my anxious thoughts.

There are both secular and faith-based meditations. The faith-based ones would have a particular Bible verse to think about and focus on during the meditation. I chose to do a mix of the two during my treatment and recovery.

I found meditation to be a good tool for calming down. I learned how to pay attention to my body and discover where I was tense. I also was able to keep relaxing images in my mind when I faced scary medical procedures.

PRAY

I did a lot of praying when I was alone in the procedure rooms. There were times that it was just the equipment and I, and I was frightened. I prayed for peace and calm so that I could get through the procedure. I had a few verses memorized that I would use as the basis of my prayers. But sometimes it was just a simple, "I'm terrified, please help." Prayer was a way for me to connect with God and give Him my raw emotions. If you have a faith background, this may be an effective way for you to walk through your fears and anxieties.

TALK & LAUGH WITH THE SUPPORT TEAM

When I wasn't in the biopsy room or waiting for a mammogram, I talked about my emotions with my support team. Sometimes this was my family and other times it was a few of my close friends. It was helpful to have people that I could call to vent to or cry with.

Consider making a list of different people you could call or talk to for different types of support. When I needed a laugh, I would go to my husband. He has a great sense of humor.

When I was checking in to my fifth biopsy, I joked with the receptionist that after this biopsy I should get a prize. Was there a special biopsy punch card I should know about? Perhaps, have 4 biopsies, get the 5th for free . . .

Dave looked at me and said, "Honey, you are the punch card!" I burst into giggles. I couldn't stop laughing. I hated biopsies so much, and he knew it. We had driven for nearly two hours to get to this location so that I could get yet another biopsy. I was done with this entire process. Laughing was therapeutic.

Think about the people in your life who are supportive. Write their names down and then reach out when you need them. These people might not be able to go into the appointments with you, but they can listen to you afterwards.

As I was walking through the biopsy phase of my treatment, I needed to slow down. I was having challenges with the procedures and the recovery. I couldn't do the normal things on my daily to-do list. As I came face to face with my weaknesses and my emotions, I realized that I had a choice to make. When I couldn't do things because I felt terrible, I could beat myself up and try to tough it out. But that didn't sit well with me.

I decided to try to accept where I was and find a way to be kind to myself. I had no idea what the next steps in this cancer journey were for me, but I wanted to figure out a way to embrace well-being and kindness towards myself. In the next chapter, I'll share in more detail what my diagnosis day looked like and how I shared the news with my loved ones.

5

DIAGNOSIS DAY

really? breast cancer for my birthday?

RESULTS DAY FINALLY ARRIVED. I was nervous about what the doctor would say, but I also felt supported because my husband would be able to take me to the appointment. I was getting my shoes on to leave when my phone rang. I saw that it was my surgeon. Why was he calling?

When I answered, he said, "I'm so sorry, but we don't have the results yet from your biopsy. Can you call the office and make an appointment for Thursday? I don't want you to come in when I don't have anything to discuss with you." I hung up and promptly fell apart.

That brief phone call from my surgeon evaporated what was left of my emotional stamina. This was my first experience with a treatment delay. It would not be my last. In this chapter, I share what it was like to get my diagnosis and what my results meant for the next steps in my treatment.

MY JOURNEY
RESULTS DAY, TAKE TWO

I had gotten through the last several days anticipating that Tuesday was *the day*. And now I had to wait another two days. Dave wouldn't be able to come with me that Thursday, so I was going to need to call in my support team.

I was devastated. But there was work to be done. I called the office and moved my appointment, then reached out to Rebekah to see if she could come with me. Thankfully, she was available.

The rest of that day was a blur of frustration, anger, fear, and powerlessness. Didn't the lab know that my life lay in the balance with these results? I was feeling dramatic and angry. I had everything all worked out and then had to change plans.

Results day, take two. Thursday. Rebekah pulled up in her van to pick me up. I had this strange sense of anticipation coupled with terror. I had a fear that I would have cancer. I had lumps in my breasts that I could feel, and those were benign. The calcifications that the radiologist had biopsied were something different and new. I didn't have a good feeling.

We arrived at the office, and she prayed for me before we walked up. We did all the normal appointment check-in tasks and tried to pass the time by talking about non-cancer things.

The surgeon arrived, greeted me, then immediately went to open my file on the computer. He turned and looked at me and said that the biopsy had revealed an area of DCIS. Rebekah wrote notes as fast as she could, the surgeon kept talking, and I just froze.

It was the day before my 42nd birthday and I was officially a cancer patient. Breast cancer was not on my birthday list, and yet it showed up. What was my life going to look like now?

The surgeon was reviewing some of the information from the report on his computer when he realized he didn't have enough information. He picked up the phone and called the radiologist. They talked for a few minutes so that he was able to get the answers he needed. He switched into surgical planning mode and was ready to get all the information he needed.

Once he hung up, we continued our conversation. He said that the initial area looked like four millimeters of non-invasive cancer. His recommendation was that I have a lumpectomy to remove the DCIS, but that I should have more tests done to have a thorough plan.

He wanted me to have more imaging done, an MRI, and he asked me to consider genetic testing. He thought that the insurance would cover the genetic testing because I was under 45 at diagnosis.

I asked him if he would be willing to get an initial surgery date on the calendar before I had the other tests done. My mom was coming into town for a month-long visit, and I thought it would be good to have her around to help me recover. Additionally, it was late September. I wanted to get the cancer out before the holidays.

He was willing to set a temporary surgery date. After the appointment, I met with his nurse to work on scheduling. We settled on a day that was a few weeks away, and then I was handed a list of things to do. I was a brand-new cancer patient, but there was work to be done.

Rebekah and I walked out of the office and collapsed on nearby chairs. I was in shock. It is a good thing that she was there because she was able to help me with the logistics. She looked through the papers and sorted out what we needed to do before she took me home. I decided to get the blood work started and then get the MRI scheduled. I needed to call the genetic counselor and schedule an appointment with my primary care doctor for surgical clearance, but I would do that when I got home.

While I was waiting for my blood work, my watch buzzed. It was my younger son, Dan. He was home alone and anxious to hear the results. I think he knew that it was not good because I was taking too long at the appointment. I texted him that I was still there but that I'd be home soon. There was no way I was going to tell him I had cancer over a text message.

Somehow, I made it through the blood work without passing out. I was in this numb state where I was trying to get through it so I could get home and collapse. Once the blood work was finished and the appointment was made for my MRI, Rebekah drove me home. It was time for me to tell my family about my diagnosis.

UNDERSTANDING PATHOLOGY
INFORMATION REVEALED FROM BIOPSY

Biopsies can reveal a lot of information that helps the surgeons make a game plan for your treatment. This initial pathology, also called the clinical pathology, is not as thorough as what will be done after surgery. Pathology reports contain vocabulary that we might not be familiar with.

I'm going to give a broad overview of what information you might get during your results call or appointment.[1]

BENIGN

Not all lesions in the breast are cancer. If the cells taken in the core-needle sample have no cancer in them, the pathology result will be benign. Your radiologist or surgeon may have a recommendation for follow-up imaging later to monitor. In some cases, these lesions might be recommended for removal, especially if they are above a certain size or cause you discomfort. Some benign breast findings that don't increase the risk of breast cancer may include: cysts, fat necrosis, fibroadenoma, fibrocystic breast changes, pseudoangiomatous stromal hyperplasia (PASH), and granular cell tumors.[2]

PRECANCEROUS OR HIGH-RISK

These findings, which might also be called *benign with upgrade potential*, are not cancer yet, but carry a higher risk of becoming cancer in the future. Depending on your pathology and risk profile, these can be monitored for changes over time, or removed. Some of these conditions may include: atypical ductal hyperplasia (ADH), atypical lobular hyperplasia (ALH), intraductal papilloma, lobular carcinoma in situ (LCIS), and phyllodes tumor.

INCONCLUSIVE

Sometimes, the core-needle biopsy doesn't reveal enough information for a pathologist to make a conclusive determination. If this is the case, the surgeon will make a recommendation for next steps. This could mean a surgical biopsy or removal via lumpectomy. In 2022, I had this result, and to read what happened, you can turn to the epilogue.

CANCER

A biopsy provides information for a conclusive cancer diagnosis. With the pathology report from the biopsy, the surgeon is able to make treatment recommendations. The initial pathology report provides a variety of information. Below is an overview of what might be included in your report:

> **Invasive and Non-Invasive.** There are two broad categories of breast cancer. There is non-invasive cancer, also called *in situ*. Those words literally mean "in place." If your cancer is *in situ* that means it hasn't invaded the surrounding tissue. If the cancer is invasive, then it has broken through the ducts and gone into the surrounding tissue.
>
> **Location.** Breast cancer can show up in multiple locations in the breast. The most common location for cancer to begin in is the milk ducts. That is where my cancer was located. I had DCIS, *ductal carcinoma in situ*. That means "non-invasive cancer located in the milk ducts." There can also be breast cancer in the lobules. This can be non-invasive, which is considered more of a pre-cancer, or invasive. There are also more rare types of breast cancer that involve the nipple or the breast tissue in between the ducts and the lobules.

Lymph Node Involvement. During the biopsy and imaging process, the medical team will try to assess whether the cancer has spread to the lymph nodes. Our lymph system moves a clear fluid, called lymph, throughout our body. We have many lymph nodes in our armpits and chest region. If breast cancer cells move into the lymph nodes, they can spread to the rest of the body through the lymphatic system.

Historically, all lymph nodes were removed as a part of breast cancer treatment. But removing all lymph nodes can lead to other serious medical problems, such as lymphedema, which is swelling in parts of the body because the lymph fluid isn't circulating freely. Recent studies have revealed that survival for early-stage patients doesn't change when lymph nodes are removed.[3]

It is important to assess if the cancer has moved into the lymph nodes so that the impacted nodes can be removed during surgery. This will reduce the risk of the breast cancer spreading outside the breast.

Hormone and HER2 Status. The initial pathology report from the biopsy can reveal the hormone status of the cancer. There are different types of breast cancer, and the pathology can determine what is "feeding" the cancer.

Breast cancer can be hormone-receptor positive. Tests will be run to see if the cancer is estrogen positive or progesterone positive. These two hormones are the most common ones that feed breast cancer. If pathology reveals that your cancer is HR (hormone-receptor) positive, then medications might be prescribed after treatment to reduce the risk of the cancer returning. I'll discuss this more in chapter 10. There is also another test that reveals HER2 status. HER2 is an acronym for human epidermal growth factor receptor two. Cancer that tests positive for this growth factor reproduces quickly.[4] Your pathology report might include notations about if your sample is HER2 positive, negative, or low.[5] If the cancer is HER2 positive, or low, the treatment plan will have special protocols.

It is possible that the cancer has no receptors. This cancer is called "triple-negative" and is usually treated with chemotherapy. Cancer can also be "triple-positive" if it has all three receptors.

Size. The imaging should have been able to determine the approximate size of the breast cancer. The size of the breast cancer will impact the surgical choices available.

The biopsy pathology will not be the final testing done on the breast cancer. Once it is removed, more testing will be done. Samples of the tumor may be sent to outside labs to determine whether radiation or chemotherapy should be recommended.

Once the surgeon has the imaging, biopsy results, and genetic testing in hand, a better plan can be made. Sometimes more imaging can result in more biopsies. I ended up needing more biopsies after my MRI, which was frustrating, but ultimately gave me enough confidence to make a surgical decision.

BREAKING THE NEWS

How much or how little you share about your personal health details is totally up to you. I have decided to be very open with my breast cancer story, but you might be more comfortable with a private journey. I found that sharing my diagnosis opened the door for others to come alongside our family and offer comfort and support.

I wasn't active on social media during the diagnosis and treatment of my breast cancer. I took a break for my mental health and decided to continue doing so during treatment. I found that being on Facebook was increasing my anxiety and distracting me from the real life happening around me. Since I wasn't updating my status online regularly, I ended up communicating through phone calls, text message, and emails to my support system. I'm glad that I kept my support circle tight. It allowed me to focus on my well-being and stay confident when I made decisions.

TELLING MY FAMILY & FRIENDS–ONE AT A TIME

Rebekah drove me home after the diagnosis appointment, and it was time to tell my family what had happened. Ideally, I could have sat them all down around a table and told them all at once. But that was not the situation of the day.

Dan, my 14-year-old, was waiting at the door for me. My husband was hours away at a work meeting, and Ken, my 16-year-old, was working the drive-thru at McDonalds. I thought about waiting until everyone got home. However, Dan is a very persistent young man. I would have been dealing with questions about my results for hours. Better to get it over with now.

I sat him down and told him that I had cancer. I told him it was small and that they had caught it early. He asked me questions about surgery and if I was going to die.

That question hit me pretty hard. What was I to say about that? We all die, so I didn't feel right about saying no, I wasn't going to die. But the prognosis so far looked pretty good. I told him that the doctors were positive about how early we caught it and that it was likely I would be okay.

After I told Dan, there were a few hours left before the rest of the family would arrive home. I sat on the couch, feeling numb and in shock, before I decided to call my parents. They were shocked. My dad, a two-time cancer survivor, took it pretty hard. When I asked him later about the call, he shared this with me:

"I felt the emotion in the empty space before she spoke. My brain was preparing for words Jennifer did not want to speak. Hearing 'Dad, I have breast cancer' from your only child was frightening and sad. As I listened to Jennifer explain her cancer diagnosis, the words 'early' and 'zero' were hopeful sounds.

"Honestly, though, on the day of her call, hope was an aspiration. I was overcome with sadness for Jennifer. I could hear her fear as she spoke, and I wanted to absorb her pain, for she was too young for this journey."[6]

After I hung up with my dad, it was time to call my mom. She was due to arrive from Hawaii for her annual visit. We were looking forward to having a great time together. Except now I had cancer. This visit was not going to be a fun one.

I had no idea how this call was going to go with her. I was surprised that she handled it as well as she did. It turns out that I had only part of the story. My mom wrote later:

"I hang up the phone and start shaking. I feel a major panic attack starting. I can barely breathe. My husband is out for the day, and I have no one around. Finally, I remember my girlfriend in New York who is almost 5 years out in her breast cancer recovery, and I call her. As soon as I hear her cheery greeting, I fall apart. Through sobs and gasping for breath, I tell her the news about my daughter. Janna helps me to calm down and then asks me a lot of questions. She assures me that my daughter is in a very good place and her chances for complete recovery are very high."[7]

I had absolutely no idea that my mom had fallen apart after my phone call with her. I had expected more emotion out of her when I told her, and was surprised that she was doing so well. It turns out she was trying to be strong for me. It was only after I completed treatment that she shared her personal struggles. I found that to be a common reaction out of my support team. I didn't always get the raw emotions from my extended family and friends.

After what seemed like hours, my husband arrived home. He walked in, looked at me, gave me a hug, and said, "How bad is it?" His eyes were filled with sadness and fear. Later, he told me that he had known that the diagnosis was positive for cancer because there had been no excited text from me to brighten up his day. Apparently, no news from me was bad news.

Not long after he got home, we headed out for a walk to try to talk things through. I told him that it had been caught early, but that there was more testing to be done. We discussed how we were feeling and the tasks that were ahead of us, as well as what kind of treatment I might need after the surgery. We were still in shock and numb.

Finally, my eldest son, Ken, arrived home from his work shift, and I was able to tell him the results. He seemed to take the news as well as could be expected, but he is much more of an internal processor. Over the next few days, I listened as he played his emotions out during his piano practice sessions. Outwardly, he had a maturity and calm, but I could hear the depth of his feelings as the music filled our home.

After I told Ken, I collapsed. It had been a long day, and I was emotionally exhausted. I didn't take the most efficient route in telling my family and friends. I remember feeling like I needed to personally deliver the news to people so that I could address their feelings and concerns one by one. In retrospect, that wasn't the best decision for my emotional stamina.

DESIGN COMMUNICATION STRATEGIES THAT DON'T EXHAUST YOU

Things will change frequently as you continue through this diagnosis and treatment path. There will be updates that will be important to share with your immediate and extended support team. Communicating updates to others can be exhausting, which I found out the hard way.

By the end of that first day, I was emotionally exhausted from all of the conversations. I was supported and loved by my family and friends, but so drained. I had received life-changing news, and rather than taking the time to understand my own feelings and care for myself, I expended a lot of energy on others. If I had it to do over again, I would have prioritized my own feelings and allowed myself the time to process before letting those outside my family know. The phone calls were draining, so gradually I developed a new strategy that allowed me to keep people updated and preserve my energy.

I had a few people who would get phone calls with important information. These were my closest family and friends. After I called them, I would take some time to write down the updates in a note on my phone. I would then copy and paste this note into an email or a text message. That way, I didn't need to rewrite the update when a friend reached out to see how I was doing. I could do a personal reply, and then paste the update right into the message.

If you are comfortable posting updates on social media, that can also be an efficient way of sharing. Doing so raises privacy issues because these updates might be more personal than you would like to share with everyone. Alternatively, there are some websites that offer password-protected options for patients to communicate with their support team. I have also seen some people share the news in a private group they establish on Facebook.

I found it emotionally exhausting to tell my diagnosis story and updates to my support team. But I wanted to keep them up to date because they were being so supportive.

OTHERS' JOURNEYS
SHARING WITH WORK

Another consideration is the timing of sharing the news with your workplace. When I was doing interviews for this book, several, but not all, of the women said that they told their supervisors right away. While you may not be able to know exactly what your treatment will be yet, you can begin to explore what your options would be for sick days, disability, family leave, and flexible working hours.

davita Had just started a new job when she found a lump. "I started my job 10/28 and diagnosed 11/20. I told my boss I was going to have a mammo due to a lump my husband found. I am pretty open and felt no need to hide it. If it was something, I would have to tell them anyway and if not, then no harm."[8]

jennifer f. "I worked up until surgery and expected to go back to work after two weeks. Given [that] my plan changed, and I was being referred for chemotherapy and radiation, I ended up being out of work for six months. I work in a correctional facility and, given my compromised immune system, it was decided that returning to work was not my best option until I finished treatments. I called my boss when I first received the diagnosis. The world was changing so quickly at that time due to the pandemic, I felt it best she knew right away so she could make the best decisions for my co-workers. I ended up on state disability, which was helpful."[9]

jill "The day I was diagnosed I was just starting my last semester of college so I was not working but attending school full-time. I ended up taking the semester off to focus on navigating treatment."[10]

betty Interviewed and was hired while undergoing chemo treatment. Didn't disclose her treatment until surgery. "With my current employer, I was already bald at the time of my interview. Luckily, my interview was over the phone. It is hard living a lie, but at the time, I didn't feel like I had the option of being truthful. I was lucky that my chemo was every three weeks on Thursday afternoon. I was on steroids the day before and after, so I was full of energy on Fridays. By the time I got home, the steroids wore off and chemo started to hit. For four months from my hire date, I would sleep from Friday till Monday morning during my chemo cycle weekend. One of my co-workers asked how I always had perfect hair. I told her it was a wig and did not explain any further. From my first day on 04/04/22 until my first surgery on 07/07/22 no one was the wiser. I am sure I could have continued not sharing the truth, but by this time I had proven my value to the company and was viewed as an asset rather than an inconvenient burden."[11]

BREAST CANCER & CHILDREN

It can be challenging to decide how much to share about your diagnosis with your children. Much of this depends on your own comfort level and the ages of your children.

If you have very young children, they might only be able to understand that mommy is sick and needs special treatment from a doctor.

If your children are in elementary school, they can be introduced to the word "cancer." This might help them understand that they can't catch it from you. There are online resources available that might be helpful as you approach the conversation. I've included some of these in the appendix. There are also children's books available that can provide other ways for you to talk to your children at a level they can understand.

Since my children were teenagers when I received the diagnosis, I chose to be very open with them. There were moments of awkwardness as I discussed my treatment. There were also a lot of conversations around the dinner table about breasts!

My two boys reacted quite differently to my diagnosis and treatment. Ken seemed to get more introverted and quiet. As I mentioned before, I sensed his emotions most clearly when he sat down at the piano and played for hours. It was as if he could escape all the chaos by letting his feelings flow into the instrument. He would also disappear for hours in his room, reading books.

On the other hand, Dan was really emotional. He would come and sit next to me on the couch and just start crying. He would tell me that he didn't want me to die. When he wasn't crying, he was angry because all of our normal routines were messed up. It was hard for me to handle his big emotions, so I would leave and hide out in my room while my husband dealt with the emotional explosions.

If you have adult children, they might be a significant help to you during your treatment. If you are comfortable, they can help you sort through treatment options and transport you to your appointments.

Cancer is a family diagnosis. I was the one going through the treatment, but my family was also walking through it. They were thinking about the possibility of my death. I had conversations with my husband about what it might look like if I died, and he needed to finish raising the boys as a widower. My kids were sorting through their feelings of fear and anger while I was going through the biopsies and treatments.

DEALING WITH OPINIONS

Once I started telling people about my diagnosis, I got an earful of other people's opinions. For the most part, I was supported and cared for as I shared. I discovered that there were many cancer survivors around me, and they were encouraging me as I was walking through the process. But sometimes conversations would start with "Well, if I were you . . ."

Here's a tip: If the sentence starts that way, run away, or change the topic!

In the beginning, I was still sorting through and processing my own emotions and treatment decisions, and I wasn't in any shape to talk through and "justify" my choices. I had no idea what was going on, and I was in no shape mentally or emotionally to deal with some of the conversations.

I discovered that I needed to gracefully exit conversations if I was getting upset. I would either find a way to change the topic or hang up the phone. Sometimes, if it was a dinner table conversation, I needed to excuse myself and go upstairs. I was emotionally charged, and no good would come from responding in anger.

MENTAL WELL-BEING
BE YOUR OWN ADVOCATE

The initial diagnosis and decision-making phase was one of the most difficult for my mental well-being. My thoughts would spin as I thought about all the different possibilities. These thoughts would lead me right down the path of anxiety.

One of the ways that I tried to address the anxiety was to learn to advocate for myself as a patient. I tried to take an active role in my treatment and recovery process by doing several things:

Ask questions. I asked a lot of questions of my doctors. I wanted to understand why they were recommending specific treatments for me.

Do research. I did a lot of research on my own to understand the treatments. I will include some of the most useful resources that I found in the appendix.

Take all my appointment time. I would take as much time as necessary to get my concerns addressed. My appointment time with them was valuable, and if I took more time than they had allocated, they could make it up another way.

Prioritize my quality of life. I prioritized my quality of life during and after my treatment. I didn't dismiss my side effects or feelings as irrelevant or invalid. I wanted to preserve as much physical wellness as possible during this treatment process. This wasn't easy because the cancer treatments were hard to cope with. The fatigue and skin peeling that I dealt with during radiation was hard. When my doctors asked me about my fatigue level, I was honest about how tired I really was.

LEARNING A NEW VOCABULARY AS PART OF OUR ADVOCACY

Cancer has its own vocabulary. As soon as that initial imaging report came back, I realized that there were a lot of words for me to learn. When I was having conversations with my surgeon, and he said a word I didn't understand, I would stop him and ask him to define the word.

After my MRI, the surgeon was going over my results with me. He was telling me that I had PASH. I looked at him in confusion. What was that, and did it need to be removed? I asked him to stop and define it for me. He told me how to spell the acronym and then told me it was benign. That was good enough for me during the appointment.

I got home and needed to find out exactly what that was. PASH is a rare benign breast condition that is sometimes detected on MRIs. It stands for pseudoangiomatous stromal hyperplasia. Well, now I knew why they used the acronym to describe it. What a mouthful! In the researching process for this book, I discovered that the National

Institute of Health has a dictionary for health terms. It is an excellent resource to use to look up unfamiliar terms.[12]

LEARNING & ADVOCACY HELP MANAGE MENTAL STRAIN

When we are first learning to drive, everything is new, and we need to exert a lot of concentration to safely get from one place to another. But as we gain more skill, the mental strain is lessened. The skills become more automatic.

This is the case even with a breast cancer diagnosis. Once we learn the language, we are better able to communicate our diagnosis with others in the community. We don't need to spend as much mental energy understanding the new language.

I would do batches of research during my diagnosis phase. I would learn everything I needed to know about PASH and then I would stop. I have enough working knowledge of the condition to explain it to someone if necessary.

The mental traffic slowed as I learned more about my diagnosis and treatment. I also felt less anxious because I understood what the doctors were talking about.

EMOTIONAL WELL-BEING

DEALING WITH STRONG EMOTIONS

I was in shock from the diagnosis for the first day or so. I made the necessary phone calls and talked to my family. I felt like I was doing pretty well with everything. That didn't last forever.

In chapter 1, I mentioned that I was in tears for most of my 42nd birthday dinner. I also fell apart regularly during church services. We would be singing a hymn with lines extolling the faithfulness of God, and the tears would begin flowing. I would stop singing because my voice was cracking. The melodies and lyrics pierced my soul. I had no idea what was next, and I was desperate to cling to my faith to get me through. Hope and fear coexisted in those moments, and crying was the overflow valve for my soul. I ended up deciding that I needed to have a pack of tissue close at hand during worship services.

Emotions can run the gamut after a cancer diagnosis. I had times when I felt like I had it together. Then I would fall apart crying or would start yelling at someone.

KEYS FOR DEALING WITH STRONG EMOTIONS

I developed coping strategies to deal with the strong emotions as they came up. These helped me sort out my feelings without yelling at my family.

> **Be aware.** The first key that I learned was to be aware of *what* I was feeling. I began to notice the physical signals when I was getting angry or anxious. I would clench my teeth and feel tightness in my chest. These were my cues to do something right away.

> **Move away.** When I felt those physical signals I needed to step away. If I was on the phone with someone, I would find a gracious way to get out of

the phone call. If I was sitting at the dinner table and the conversation was getting difficult, I would excuse myself and go up to my room.

This was not something that I usually needed to do. Generally, I have been able to stay calm during family dinners. But my kids were having a hard time dealing with the cancer. Dan, in particular, was scared and angry. His feelings would come out at dinner, and I was unable to have a rational conversation with him. Thankfully, my husband was able to listen and talk with him through most of his emotional outbursts.

I would walk away and take some time to figure out how I was feeling. Sometimes, I would journal my thoughts, and other times I would pray or meditate. The goal was to try to bring my emotional temperature down from boiling to simmering.

Adjust. The next thing I would do was to try to adjust my perspective on the situation. I would try to identify exactly why I was getting angry and then see the conversation from the other person's point of view. If I could acknowledge how scary my diagnosis was for my family, I could better understand their emotions.

Sometimes, I would have a conversation with a loved one to try to help them understand where I was coming from. This usually went better when I had calmed down. We could have a much more productive conversation when I wasn't yelling or crying!

WHEN TO GET PROFESSIONAL HELP

It is completely normal to be feeling anxious and worried after getting a cancer diagnosis.[13] However, if you are finding that you are unable to do the normal activities, please talk to your medical team. There are trained psychologists who work specifically with cancer patients. This specialty is called onco-psychology.

Your family might be struggling as well and could benefit from seeking out help either in the form of a support group or therapy. Cancer is a challenging illness to deal with, so if things are getting overwhelming, please reach out for support. Talk to your doctors and get referrals for mental health care.

One of the biggest challenges to my emotional and mental well-being was the decision of which surgery to have. Would I have a lumpectomy plus radiation, or would a mastectomy be a better choice? In order to make an informed decision, the imaging needed to be complete, the biopsies had to finish, and the results from my genetic testing needed to get back from the lab. In the next chapter, I will provide an overview of some of the surgical choices for breast cancer treatment and share how I made my decision.

6

MAKING A SURGICAL GAME PLAN

IN THE UNITED STATES prior to 1998, reconstruction after a mastectomy could be considered a cosmetic procedure. This meant that insurance companies could approve a mastectomy but not approve the rebuilding of a woman's breast.

The U.S. Women's Health and Cancer Rights Act of 1998[1] provided federal protection to women after breast cancer surgery. This law is also sometimes called "Janet's Law" because the crusade began with a 32-year-old breast cancer patient, Janet Franquet, and her surgeon. Janet had required reconstruction after her mastectomy, but her insurance plan denied coverage stating that it was a cosmetic procedure. The argument was that the breast is not a medically required appendage and didn't require replacing. Her surgeon, Dr. Todd Wider, did the procedure for free and then began a national crusade to end this type of insurance denial for patients. The law passed in October 1998.

Women are now allowed to choose reconstruction, if desired, and have it covered by insurance. Additionally, if a woman decides to remain flat, breast prosthetics are covered by insurance. While this law doesn't take care of all costs associated with breast cancer care, it does provide guidelines so that insurance must cover the reconstruction as well as the cancer removal.

In this chapter, I will discuss the surgical and reconstruction options available to breast cancer patients as well as discuss the role that genetic testing might play in the decision-making process.

MY JOURNEY
MASTECTOMY OR LUMPECTOMY

Do I remove part of my breast or all of it? That was the question facing me after my diagnosis with DCIS. I asked my surgeon if we could do active surveillance and just keep an eye on things for a while. I really hoped to avoid surgery. My surgeon didn't recommend that for me. He did mention that there was an ongoing trial which was testing to see if observation would be a viable choice in DCIS patients, but I wasn't a candidate for the study.[2] I was facing surgery.

Some cancer diagnoses allow for us to choose between the surgeries. Suprisingly, this can feel more overwhelming because we feel the weight of making the "right" choice. I felt that tension as I walked through my decision-making process.

The excellent news is that both a lumpectomy and a mastectomy are highly effective at removing the cancer.

Both surgeries work. On the other hand, no surgery completely eliminates the risk of getting breast cancer again.

Recurrence either in the remaining breast tissue, or elsewhere in the body, is possible with each choice. There are some choices that will lower the risk of recurrence more than others, but no surgical choice can completely eliminate the risk.

This was an important factor in my decision-making process. If there was some way for me to ensure that I would never get breast cancer again, I would make that choice. But there isn't a surgery that can do that. So, as I examined each surgery, I decided to focus on how I wanted to treat this instance of cancer. It might come back, and I might need to make a different choice in the future. I needed to stay in the moment and choose the surgery that made the most sense for this diagnosis.

In the next section, I will delve into the two types of surgeries, mastectomy and lumpectomy, and discuss the possible reconstruction options.

OPTION
MASTECTOMY

Depending on the extent of the breast cancer found, this surgery to remove one or both breasts might be the only option offered to you. There have been many advances in this surgery that allow women to choose from a variety of reconstruction types or to remain flat.

A mastectomy may include multiple procedures and surgeries to achieve the desired cosmetic appearance. A breast surgeon typically works with a plastic surgeon or reconstruction specialist to design a specific strategy for each patient. These providers work together to remove the cancer and then reconstruct your new breast.[3]

During a mastectomy, the surgeon will remove the breast tissue and also examine the surrounding lymph nodes to see which ones appear cancerous. Additionally, there may be pathology run on certain nodes to determine the extent of the cancer spread. Once the desired amount of tissue is removed, the reconstruction process can begin.

TYPES OF RECONSTRUCTION

Immediate, or Direct to Implants. In some cases, the surgeons will be able to perform the mastectomy and then place implants at the same time. This can minimize subsequent surgeries and allow the patient to wake up with the reconstruction complete.

Expanders. If going direct to implants isn't an option, then surgeons may place expanders in the breast. An expander is an empty breast implant that has a fill valve. Over the course of several office visits, these expanders will be filled with saline until the breast reaches the desired size.

Expanders can be placed over or under the chest muscles. Before surgery, take some time to discuss which option will be used for your surgery.

Once the expanders have been completely filled, another surgery will be scheduled to get the permanent implants. This is called an *exchange surgery*.

Flap Reconstruction. Some surgeons offer a reconstruction using your own fat tissue. This fat can be taken from the stomach, buttocks, or thighs. The fat can then be placed into the breast. These have different names based on the location of the tissue being moved. One of the most common types of flap reconstruction is called DIEP. In this surgery, the tissue comes from the stomach.

This option is like getting liposuction in one area and getting a breast reconstruction. These flap reconstructions are complicated procedures and not all breast surgeons can do them. Also, they typically require multiple surgeries to achieve the desired appearance.

Flap reconstructions allow women to have reconstructed breasts that look more natural because the breasts are constructed of natural tissue instead of implants. Additionally, there are no implants that might need monitoring or replacing.

If you choose this option, check your insurance coverage for the specific procedures you will be having. While reconstruction is protected under WHCRA, the types of reconstruction covered may vary.

Going Flat. Another option is to skip the reconstruction altogether. Many women are choosing this option to avoid implants or multiple surgeries. If this option is of interest to you, I would recommend researching the option of having an aesthetic flat closure.[4] This is a reconstructive procedure that rebuilds the shape of the chest wall after a single or double mastectomy. The skin will be smoothed out so that the chest wall is nearly flat. An aesthetic flat closure avoids skin folds, sometimes called "dog ears," which can happen after the removal of the breast tissue.

Goldilocks Mastectomy. This surgery is in between full reconstruction and an aesthetic flat closure. A Goldilocks mastectomy uses the remaining skin and tissue to create a small breast mound. This option allows a woman to retain some breast shape without going through a full reconstruction. The size of the reconstructed breast mound will be determined by how much available skin and tissue the patient has after the appropriate amount of tissue has been removed.[5]

Single Mastectomy. If the cancer is located in only one breast, you may have an option to choose a single mastectomy. This option allows you to retain feeling and sensation in the non-cancerous breast. Reconstruction, if desired, would then only be done on the breast removed.

MASTECTOMY: THINGS TO CONSIDER

The physical recovery from a mastectomy varies greatly from patient to patient. There are many different factors in place that make it difficult to predict whose recovery will progress quickly, and whose will take more time. A general guideline for recovery is between four and six weeks, if things are going smoothly. Recovery challenges, such as infection, can set the recovery process back. A mastectomy is a major surgery, and the recovery will take time.

Continuing to get the recommended screenings is important because it is impossible to remove all the breast tissue in a mastectomy. Since some tissue will remain, there is a possibility of breast cancer returning in the remaining tissue.

As I was doing research on mastectomies, one of the most startling things I learned is that in most cases the breasts become numb after surgery. When the breast is removed in surgery, the nerves in the area are cut. This means the reconstructed breast will lose all feeling. This can present a significant quality of life issue for women. In fact, numbness was the primary reason that I decided not to choose a mastectomy.

Breast surgeons are aware of this challenge facing women and have developed techniques to preserve breast sensation.[6] Sensation-preserving mastectomies are not standard practice as of this writing, so if this is something you are seeking, I recommend asking your surgeon about options available to you.

Nipples are usually removed during a mastectomy, unless the procedure is a nipple-sparing mastectomy. Once reconstruction is completed, nipples can be added with a variety of techniques. Nipple tattoos can be done by tattoo artists, or a three-dimensional nipple can be done as part of a surgical procedure. Surgeons generally recommend waiting several months after the last reconstructive surgery to add nipples. This allows the breasts to heal and settle so that the nipple placement is precise.

If this all seems overwhelming and too much to process, I can relate. There is a lot that goes into making a surgical decision. Thankfully, reconstruction decisions can be made months or years after surgery. I spoke to women who had initially decided to go flat but then opted for reconstruction later. There were also women who decided to have their implants removed to go flat or have a flap procedure done.

Mastectomies have progressed significantly since the very first one was performed. Modern mastectomies offer women a range of choices for reconstruction. Women can also choose to forgo reconstruction and have an aesthetically pleasing flat chest.

OPTION
LUMPECTOMY

In 1985, research revealed that lumpectomy plus radiation was an effective treatment for early-stage breast cancer.[7] This research allowed for a lumpectomy to be a viable and effective choice for patients. A lumpectomy can also be called a *partial mastectomy* or *breast-conserving surgery*. At my initial diagnosis, my breast surgeon recommended a lumpectomy because it was less invasive than a mastectomy and equally effective at removing the cancer.

The advantage of a lumpectomy is that it removes the cancer while preserving the rest of the breast. It is a less invasive surgery, and the recovery time is usually much faster than with a mastectomy. Throughout my diagnosis process, I hoped that I would be able to have my DCIS removed with a lumpectomy because it was so small.

Cosmetic Results. During a lumpectomy, a surgeon can use a variety of techniques to have the breasts look as natural as possible after the procedure. Some of these include hiding the incisions so that they aren't as noticeable. My surgeon did a technique called flap rearrangement on one of the lumps he removed. This technique preserved the natural shape of my breast even after the tissue was removed.

Some cosmetic challenges after a lumpectomy might include dips or bulges in the area of the removal or a difference in sizes between the two breasts. Another possible issue is that, due to tissue removal, one of the nipples might point in a different direction after the lumpectomy.

I recommend discussing these cosmetic issues with your surgeon before the procedure. Initially, I was uncomfortable talking about the potential appearance of my post-lumpectomy breasts. Whenever I was filled with discomfort, I remembered a conversation that I had with another breast cancer patient. Janna had chosen a lumpectomy but didn't discuss any reconstructive options that might have been available to her during surgery. She ended up needing to wait almost a year to have the lumpectomy reconstruction completed. She encouraged me to bring up any concerns about my cosmetic results *before* my surgery so that I had the appropriate surgical team in place.

Janna's words echoed in my mind as I mustered the strength to discuss my cosmetic results with my breast surgeon. On one of my phone conversations with him,

I was practically in tears while I was asking him if my breasts would be pretty after he was done.

It was worth it to push through the discomfort, even if my words were emotional and raw. I was relieved after having the uncomfortable cosmetic conversation with him.

These were a few of the things I discussed with my surgeon:

- Location of incisions
- Preserving my breast shape
- Nipple direction—I wanted them still facing front
- Size of scars
- Minimization of scars

As I mentioned above, if the amount of tissue being removed is large, there is a possibility to do reconstruction. This can happen at the same time as surgery, or it can be done later to address any issues that may occur after the initial lumpectomy.

Clean Margins. This is an important part of a successful lumpectomy. The surgeon will aim to remove the cancer and a surrounding portion of tissue that doesn't have cancer. This is known as *clean margins*. Depending on your diagnosis, clean, or clear, margins might be a standard of "no ink on tumor" or a specific number of millimeters of normal tissue around the cancer.[8]

A clean margin is associated with a lower risk of recurrence. Unfortunately, not all lumpectomies are performed with clean margins during the first time. If the margins are not clean, then another surgery, called a re-excision, may be necessary. Statistics say that re-excision rates run at around 25 percent.[9] But this percentage is not across the board. Surgeons who perform a lot of lumpectomies tend to have much lower re-excision rates.

A surgeon's re-excision rate is a very important consideration. I highly recommend asking your breast surgeon what her rate of re-excision is. There are techniques that can be done during surgery that aid in achieving clean margins.[10]

I didn't know that re-excision was so common when I was choosing to do a lumpectomy. I didn't ask my surgeon about his re-excision rates before surgery. Recently, I had an appointment with him, and asked. He said that his re-excision rate was 8 percent. This is extremely low, and I was impressed. When I asked him why it was so low, he told me that it was because he worked with a pathology team during the surgery to see if he removed the cancer with clean margins. This pathology was done in real time, and I was able to see in the notes that his first removal didn't have clean margins, but the second one did.

REDUCTION & LIFT WITH LUMPECTOMY

This is another option to remove the cancer and also enhance the appearance of the remaining breast tissue. This surgery is called an *oncoplastic reduction*. It removes the cancer along with additional breast tissue. This technique can help the breast surgeon create a uniform appearance for the breasts, and it can also reduce some of the sagging that comes with age. If you are well-endowed and have considered a breast reduction in the past, it may be worthwhile for you to discuss this option with your surgeon. I have spoken to many women who have chosen this surgery and are very happy with the results. With a oncoplastic reduction, clean margins are not usually as big a concern because more breast tissue is being removed.

LUMPECTOMY: THINGS TO CONSIDER

A lumpectomy is usually performed as an outpatient surgery, and the recovery is about two to three weeks. However, this may be delayed if there are challenges clearing the margins. It is a much less involved surgery than a mastectomy. Lymph nodes will be tested if your cancer is invasive, and the impacted nodes can be removed during the surgery. If radiation is recommended after a lumpectomy, it can be started once your surgeon clears you. I started radiation about a month after my lumpectomy.

GENETIC TESTING

In 2013, Angelina Jolie went public in an op-ed for the *New York Times*. After testing positive for the BRCA gene, she decided to undergo a "contralateral preventative mastectomy." Her mother, grandmother, and aunt had all died of cancer. In choosing a mastectomy, Jolie was able to dramatically reduce her risk of developing breast cancer. Her story has had a profound impact on cancer treatment.

The number of women choosing to undergo this type of procedure has increased significantly all around the world. Scientists have studied and named this phenomenon "The Angelina Jolie Effect."[11]

Despite her passionate plea that all women get tested for the BRCA gene, it still isn't standard practice to undergo genetic testing for a breast cancer diagnosis. This is because only about one in ten breast cancers are linked to a genetic mutation. However, individuals who are carriers of specific mutations do have a significantly increased risk of developing breast cancer.

Genetic counseling and testing may be a part of your diagnosis process, especially if you meet certain criteria. Testing may be indicated if you are under 45, have family members with reproductive cancers (ovarian, prostate, breast, uterine), or are a member of certain ethnic groups. People of Ashkenazi Jewish or Eastern European heritage carry the BRCA gene in a higher percentage than other ethnicities.[12] I have included a chart from the CDC in the chapter references that can help you determine what your personal genetic risk may be for developing cancer.[13]

Genetic testing can help patients and medical teams make a more thorough plan for treatment. I decided to have genetic testing done to make sure I was choosing the most effective surgery for me.

MY EXPERIENCE WITH GENETIC COUNSELING

To get the genetic testing done, I needed to make an appointment with the genetic counselor. She would meet with me, go over my family history, and determine if I met the insurance criteria for genetic testing. Since only about 10 percent of breast cancers are believed to be caused by genetic variations, insurance companies limit their coverage of these tests to individuals who fall into a higher risk category.

Before I had the appointment with the genetic counselor, I received a thick packet in the mail. I needed to fill in a thorough family history which would give the geneticist information about previous cancers. There were several times that I needed to call my parents to get the information correct.

If you are adopted and are seeking information about your blood relatives for these forms, you might consider asking your adoptive parents if they received any family history from the adoption agency. Age can be used as a determining factor for insurance coverage in the absence of a family history due to adoption.[14]

I filled out all the forms as best as I could before the appointment so that I would be prepared. I was thrilled that my mom was in town and would be able to come with me. She would be able to answer any questions about her side of the family and take notes for me.

The genetic counseling appointment was one of my favorite appointments—and not just because I got to keep my shirt on. I enjoyed talking with the geneticist about the family history, watching her fill out the genetic family tree, and getting my questions answered about what testing might reveal about my genetic makeup. While I didn't have a lot of breast cancer in my family, I did have family members with prostate cancer on both my maternal and paternal sides, and I was of Norwegian descent, which placed me at a higher risk for a variant.

My family history and my age met the criteria for insurance coverage for genetic testing. Ultimately, the question of testing was placed into my lap. Did I want to proceed? It was a resounding *yes*. I wanted to know if I was carrying genetic variants that increased my risk. Maybe that was the reason I got cancer.

I was offered three different levels of genetic testing. One was a test that assessed variants linked to breast cancer, and the other two increased the number of genes tested. I decided on the most thorough panel, which tested 77 genes. This was my one opportunity to get a window into my genetic makeup, and I wanted to have as many answers as possible.

I didn't need to leave the room for the blood draw, which surprised me. I was sitting in the chair in the examination room and my mom was sitting at the edge of the exam table, where she had been during the appointment taking notes. Before the nurse got started, I warned her that I had a tendency to pass out during blood draws. She didn't seem too worried and went out to grab a pillow to put on my lap. I looked at her quizzically and said, "Shouldn't I get up on the table to lie down?"

"No, you'll be fine," was her response. She and my mom chatted about how they both did totally fine during blood draws. I felt the tourniquet go around my arm and then the cotton feeling entered my eardrums. A warm flush came up over my body and I felt the familiar sense of the shades closing around my eyes. I slumped over the pillow as my arm ached with the pain of the tight elastic band around my arm.

I felt the needle come out of my arm after what felt like an eternity. I weakly asked, "Could I please have some juice?"

I raised my head, opened my eyes, and tried to shake off the lingering sensations. I saw my mom's eyes fill with worry, fear, and helplessness. "Are you okay?" she asked.

"I told you I might pass out!" The nurse returned with the juice box and asked me how I was doing. I told her I might need a bit of time to feel up to leaving the room and thanked her for the juice. I'm pretty sure if there was a second blood test needed, I would have been able to lie down on the table. Neither my mom nor the nurse had believed I would pass out. Thankfully, I didn't fall onto the floor.

My samples were sent to the lab, and it would be a few weeks until I had the results. There was a rush placed on the portion of the test centered on the breast cancer genes, and I hoped that it would be back before my surgery.

WHY I CHOSE A LUMPECTOMY

The original recommendation from my surgeon was to have a lumpectomy to remove my DCIS. However, he wanted to do thorough imaging and recommended genetic counseling so that we could have as much information as possible.

The genetic testing took a few weeks to complete, even though we had asked for a rush to be put on it. Additionally, I needed to have three more biopsies after my MRI.

It was really hard to endure the waiting and the extra biopsies. But my surgeon continued to encourage me that my DCIS was not an emergency. There was time to be thorough so that I only needed to undergo one surgery. He didn't want me to choose a lumpectomy only to find out I was BRCA positive. I was grateful for his words of wisdom and his thoroughness.

I was in the car, on my way to a biopsy, when the phone rang. It was my genetic counselor. She was excited to tell me that I had tested negative for the genetic mutations. I was absolutely giddy on the phone with her. I told her that she was giving me the first bit of good news in a long time. She shared my enthusiasm and was happy to have been able to reach me before I went into my biopsies that week.

I hung up the phone and felt a huge sigh of relief. If the additional biopsies were benign, I would be able to have the lumpectomy. I really didn't want to have a mastectomy unless it was medically necessary. My DCIS was the size of a grain of rice. I wasn't ready to say goodbye to my breasts over a small malignancy.

When my additional biopsies came back benign, it further cemented my decision. I would choose a lumpectomy plus radiation. It seemed to make sense for me. My recovery would be quicker, and I could keep my breasts. I would need to make sure to keep up with regular scans, but I would rather get a mammogram a couple of times a year than undergo a major surgery plus reconstruction.

If my breast cancer comes back, I will need to revisit my surgical choices. However, I needed to stay in the moment and treat the cancer that I had. Dwelling in "what ifs" added to my anxiety.

OTHERS' JOURNEYS
SURGICAL DECISIONS

There are so many factors that impact our surgical choices. While I decided on a lumpectomy, that may not be an option for you. You may prefer a mastectomy. Here are stories of other breast cancer survivors and how they made their surgical choices.

As I was reading over each of these stories, I was struck by a few things. While these women all had breast cancer, they each opted for a different surgical choice. Breast cancer is not one single disease with one correct treatment option. There are many factors that can impact our decisions. These women looked at the risks and decided on the best option for them and their stage in life.

jennifer f. Bilateral mastectomy/no reconstruction yet. "Given my genetic test results and the high chances of recurrence, I opted for a bilateral mastectomy. I had hoped for immediate reconstruction, but due to COVID-19 restrictions, my medical provider did not want me to be hospitalized overnight . . . I do plan to pursue reconstruction in the future and am changing medical providers to do so. I have become more comfortable with my new body over the last six months and would be okay remaining flat should reconstruction continue to prove not to be my best option."[15]

lillian Single mastectomy with reconstruction. "I chose SMX (single mastectomy) over DMX (double mastectomy) because no genetic [variant] was found. I had no choice. I had a 2.1 cm IDC (invasive ductal carcinoma) and 9cm DCIS (ductal carcinoma in situ), which was more than half of my breast."[16]

noelle Bilateral mastectomy with immediate reconstruction. "I wanted to do everything possible to reduce my risk of developing cancer on the right side as well, so I decided to remove both breasts. While implants were not my first option, I was not a candidate for a DIEP Flap, but I knew mentally, I could not go flat. Which is funny because my entire life I had hate(d) my breasts and always just wanted them gone. Well, now that cancer was taking them from me, it helped me realize they are such a huge part of my identity as a woman."[17]

davita Mastectomy with immediate DIEP flap surgery. "I have the PALB2 gene (see appendix for resources on genes linked to breast cancer). It didn't impact my decision because I made the decision already to have a DMX (double mastectomy) due to fear of recurrence. Then, after I got my results, my genetic counselor and my doctors said we made the best choice, and had that not been the choice, they would have pushed me to do it . . . Some deciding factors for me on DIEP (flap reconstruction) vs. implants: I did not want to leave the hospital flat or with expanders; I didn't want my breast to feel cold all the time, a common implant issue; I did not want to have to have another surgery down the road to exchange them because they only last so long. Implant sickness is common among breast cancer patients, so I wanted to avoid that."[18]

sheena Goldilocks Mastectomy. "When a mastectomy became the only option, I struggled with losing my breasts and going flat or even concave with no reconstruction or doing extensive surgeries to form new breasts with implants or using my own fat from another area.

I despaired and delayed my surgery because I could not come to terms with any of these options. Then I found out about Goldilocks mastectomy (and its variations with slightly different scar patterns) that offered an appealing middle choice. I was a saggy B or C cup size to begin with, and I described what I wanted to my surgeon as a "man chest" because that was realistically all that was possible for me. Still, I was relieved that my results look feminine on me."[19]

MENTAL WELL-BEING
OWNING YOUR SURGICAL CHOICE

There can be real decision fatigue and anxiety when facing a surgical choice. Other people in your life might have opinions about which surgery you should get. They might begin conversations with words like, "Well, if I were you, I would . . ."

I found that line of conversation to be very hard to handle, especially since I was so emotionally exhausted from the diagnosis process. I like to please everyone, so being an advocate for my decision was difficult. I learned that I needed to own my surgical decision and let others have their opinions. They were not walking in my shoes and weren't facing a surgical choice.

If the surgeon is offering you an option between a lumpectomy or a mastectomy, this means that both surgeries are medically valid. Then the decision moves into the realm of personal choice. Also, the choice about what type of reconstruction doesn't need to be made right away. Jennifer F. decided to do the bilateral mastectomy and then wait to make a reconstruction decision. I have also spoken with women who have decided later on to have their implants removed and go flat or have a flap procedure done. I was comfortable with a lumpectomy for this incidence of breast cancer, but I remain open to another surgical choice if I have a recurrence.

Once I decided on a lumpectomy, I felt a huge weight lift off my shoulders. I stopped researching and second-guessing my decision. I was comfortable with my choice, and I was able to move on to preparing for surgery.

EMOTIONAL WELL-BEING
ANGER & FRUSTRATION ABOUT BREAST CANCER

I was surprised at how emotional I got when I thought about having surgery on my breasts. My breasts were a part of me that I took for granted. I enjoyed wearing pretty bras to support them. Now I was making decisions that would change them forever.

There were times I was angry that I was facing these choices in my early 40s. I had no genetic variants, and I didn't have a lot of the risk factors associated with getting breast cancer at this age. I was really afraid about what I would look like after surgery. Would my sex life ever be the same?

I found that once I made a surgical decision, my emotions got more centered. I was thankful that I would be able to have a lumpectomy. I began to shift my focus to preparing for surgery day.

As the surgery day drew near, I began to have new fears. Would I wake up from the anesthesia? I had never gone under before, and I had no idea what to expect. I was terrified about the pain and worried about my recovery. In the week that led up to my surgery I tried to enjoy the last few days with my mom and get as ready as I could. Time sped by as I took care of the final appointments and checked items off my very long to-do list. In the next chapter, I will share how I prepared myself and the home for my upcoming surgery.

7

PREPARATION FOR SURGERY

so many things to do

THE WARM WATER FLOWED over my head, and I breathed in the scent of my rose soap. I blinked my eyes open and looked at my filthy shower. "Ugh, this is not relaxing," was my next thought. "I had better do something about this grime before my surgery." Shower cleaning is my least favorite chore, but I knew that it wasn't going to get done while I was recovering. I rinsed off and added that chore to my ever-expanding list of things to do before surgery day.

There are many things to do to get ready for surgery. These logistics can be a lot to focus on, and if not addressed, can mean a surgical delay or cancellation. In this chapter, I will detail some of the ways that I prepared for surgery so that things went as smoothly as possible.

MY JOURNEY
DELAYED SURGERY MAKES FOR CHANGES IN THE PLAN

After my initial diagnosis, I had my surgeon put a tentative surgery date on the calendar. It was right in the middle of my mom's planned visit to our home, and I was grateful she would be there to help us out as I recovered. Everything was proceeding nicely, one step at a time. I had cancer, but we had a plan.

And then I got my MRI results. As I shared in chapter 3, I needed additional biopsies after my Breast MRI. Instead of facing a surgery on October 16, as I'd thought, I was now facing a delay. And since one of the findings was in my lymph nodes, I was terrified that I would need additional surgery or treatments.

As I was emotionally processing this delay, I also needed to make some practical adjustments to my planning. Would we leave the boys at home alone while I was having my lumpectomy? I didn't know when my surgery would occur, but I was pretty sure that my mom's visit was going to be finished by the time we got all the results. When I wasn't worrying about the logistics, I was worrying about what the doctors might find during the biopsies.

I had already taken care of all my pre-surgical appointments when I thought my surgery would be on the 16th. But with the delay, would I need to get all of those tests run again? My mind was spinning, my emotions were heightened, and I felt extremely overwhelmed. It was time to open up my notebook and write everything down so I could sort through the revised situation.

BEFORE SURGERY DAY

MAKE A WORKING TO-DO LIST

I recommend making a list of things to do before surgery as soon as you finalize a surgical plan and a date. If things end up changing, as they did for me, you can revisit the list and see what you've already done, and add new items as needed to your working to-do list. A few days before surgery, review that list and make any last-minute adjustments or purchases. The night before, pack your bag so that you don't need to do that the morning of surgery.

PRE-SURGERY MEDICAL APPOINTMENTS & REQUIREMENTS

Before a surgery, many appointments and tests will need to be completed. These will vary from patient to patient. After my surgical planning appointment, which took place a few weeks before my surgery, my surgeon gave me a list of things to get done before the surgery and told me exactly how to get the required information to him. All this information was on a sheet of paper he handed me at our surgical planning appointment. Here are a few things that might be on that list:

> **Blood Work.** This needs to be completed within a specific window of time to be valid. Make sure you know what that window is. In my case, it was within 30 days. This was important because my surgery was delayed. I ended up repeating my blood work just to make sure it was valid for my surgery.
>
> **Clearance from Primary Care Doctor.** I needed to make an appointment to see my primary care

doctor. She listened to my lungs, asked me some questions, and then faxed her approval over to my surgeon.

Chest X-ray. I had this done during my appointment with my primary care doctor. I wasn't sure how these results would be sent over to my surgeon because it was done at a different medical group, so I asked for a copy of the imaging results before I left the office. The radiology tech was able to make a CD of the images for me.

EKG. My primary care doctor ordered this test for me. It took longer to set up the little receptors all over my body than to run the test.

COVID-19 Test. Your hospital or surgery center may have you take a coronavirus test. Each center has a different set of requirements for quarantine or self-isolation after this test is completed. I would make sure you know what the rules are several weeks before surgery. If you are required to self-isolate, then you will need to make sure to complete the other pre-surgery tasks before the period of self-isolation.

INFORMATION TO GATHER BEFORE SURGERY

Medications to Pick Up or Stop Taking. I recommend talking about medications during your pre-surgical appointment. I asked my surgeon what medications he would prescribe for me after surgery.

I was especially concerned with pain management. I asked him what he usually prescribed and when we would get those prescriptions. He told me he would write a prescription for Tylenol with codeine for pain, an anti-nausea medication that could be taken with the pain medicine as needed, and perhaps an antibiotic. I would need the antibiotic if I came out of the surgery with surgical drains. Since he didn't know if I would need the antibiotic, the prescriptions would be given to my husband on the day of surgery.

Additionally, we discussed medications to avoid prior to surgery. These included common pain medicines like ibuprofen, aspirin, and Aleve. Make sure to tell your surgeon about all the medications and herbal supplements you take on a regular basis so that you can pause anything necessary.

Location of Lumps to Be Removed. Make sure to discuss and confirm with your surgeon exactly what will be removed and where those lumps are located on your breast. I had several benign lesions in my left breast, and the surgeon wanted to remove the largest one. I had him point out, on my breast, exactly where the two areas were. I knew where the DCIS was and where the benign fibroadenoma was. In the next chapter, I'll share the full story about what happened the day of surgery when the radiologist almost marked the wrong finding with the localizing wire. Know the exact location of the lumps to be removed before you leave the appointment.

ADMINISTRATIVE TASKS

In addition to the medical tasks above, there will be a variety of administrative tasks that may need to be done before your surgery. These can help avoid insurance or logistical issues that could potentially delay your surgery or incur extra costs.

Deliver imaging to the surgery center. I needed to hand deliver my imaging to the hospital before my surgery. The hospital was not in the same network as my medical group and would be unable to view the mammogram and ultrasound images in a shared online portal. There was no way to transmit them electronically. So, I needed to pick up a CD from my imaging center and drive it down to the women's center where the localization procedure would be performed.

Verify the hospital is in-network. This is important! If your surgery is performed at an out-of-network hospital, you may incur additional costs after surgery. At the time of my surgery, our local hospital in Santa Clarita was not in-network. My surgery needed to be done in another location where my doctor had credentials and my insurance was accepted. This was not convenient, but it avoided extra costs.

Schedule your follow-up appointment. During your pre-surgical visit, I would recommend asking your surgeon when he would like to see you for your follow-up visits. Then make that appointment before you leave the office so that it is on your calendar.

HOME & FAMILY MANAGEMENT

In addition to the many medical things on your to-do list, it is good to think about things that are important for you to take care of in the home and with your family before surgery. This might mean thinking about where your children will be while you are in surgery or who might walk your dogs for you. Here are a few of the things that I thought of before my lumpectomy:

Clean the home or have it cleaned. You'll have physical restrictions after surgery, so have the house as clean as you would like it before the surgery date. I was thankful I cleaned the shower before my lumpectomy because it was nice to recover in a clean space.

Plan care for your children. Think about what care your children will need during your surgery day—for example, rides to and from school or care at home. These tasks might provide a nice way for a grandparent or family member to give constructive help on surgery day.

If you don't have family nearby, you could ask a close friend or neighbor or hire a sitter for the day. Our friends, Scott and Judee, who live down the street, offered to watch our kids after school on my surgery day. Once my sons finished their lessons for the day, they walked over to Scott and Judee's house and spent time with them. My sons were old enough to stay home alone during my surgery, but I was uncomfortable with the thought of them not having a trusted adult around to talk to during the day.

Arrange care for pets. We decided to send our dogs to our dog sitter's home for a few days after my surgery. Our beagles are wonderful, but they bark a lot and sleep on the bed with us. I didn't want to risk them pulling out a surgical drain or jumping up and hitting my chest. I also wanted to have the option to sleep in and relax.

Having the dogs away for a few days allowed my family to ease into recovery mode. If that isn't an option for you, then consider who will take over the walking, poop, and noise patrol during your surgical recovery.

Plan meals after surgery. If you are going home on the same day as your surgery, you will likely be hungry. I was really excited to eat after a long day of fasting. Think ahead about what might be easy to eat. I wouldn't recommend planning anything too spicy. I stuck with a relatively bland diet on the day of surgery because I wasn't sure how my stomach would react after the anesthesia. Since anesthesia slows down your digestive tract, making sure to have food that is high in fiber and drinking water can get things moving and prevent constipation.

Think about a companion for your partner during surgery. Dave and I talked about this before my surgery day. I didn't want him waiting alone, but I wasn't sure who he would want to be with while I was in surgery. This was a pretty personal decision for him, especially since I wasn't going to be awake for it! I brought the idea up to him on a walk one day, not sure what he would say. I was relieved and touched to learn that his friend, Dale, had already volunteered to drive out. Dale stayed with Dave until I woke up from surgery. Having an extra person in the waiting room might be tricky with COVID-19 protocols, but it is something worth talking to your partner about before the surgery.

SURGERY DAY
CREATING A PLAN

It was one thing to have a list of things to do before surgery, but what time did I need to leave the house? How would I remember what to bring? I needed to create a plan so that I could think clearly as I dealt with the pre-surgery nerves.

TIME MANAGEMENT

I wanted to make sure that I wasn't panicked as I headed to the hospital. We live near Los Angeles, and heavy traffic is a reality. I tend to arrive at things early because I overestimate the driving time. Since this was going to be a long day, I wanted to arrive on time but not too early.

I decided to work backward from my arrival time. I estimated the travel time, then picked a reasonable time to leave. I allocated some time to get the car packed with the things that I would need during and after surgery. I put as much information as I could on the calendar so that everyone in the family was on the same page.

WHAT TO PACK FOR SURGERY DAY

Begin with the guidelines from your surgeon. I needed to bring a top that buttoned or zipped in front and a front-close bra because I would have difficulty lifting my arms over my head. I didn't need to bring that much with me because I was planning on going home that night. If you are staying in the hospital longer, you might want to bring more items in your bag.

Useful Items

- Loose, front-close top
- Comfortable pants that are easy to put on
- Front-close bra
- Non-slip socks
- Underwear
- Toothbrush/other toiletry items
- Communication tools (phone or tablet)
- Snacks for the car
- A pillow for the seatbelt—your surgeon will give you specific instructions for this. I wasn't allowed to use a shoulder belt for a few weeks.
- Water for the car ride (after the surgery)
- A bucket or bin for the car, in case you get nauseous on the ride.
- A blanket to keep you warm in the car.

STAYING IN TOUCH

On surgery day, there may be some people who would love to get updates on how things are going. In my case, that meant keeping my sons in the loop with text messages. Before I left for surgery, I created a group chat with my neighbors, Scott and Judee, my husband, and my sons. This gave Dave one chat thread to update with the progress on my surgery. It was worth it to take some time to think about who I wanted to keep updated.

THINKING AHEAD FOR AFTER SURGERY

As much as I wanted the surgery to be the finish line of this cancer journey, I knew that I needed to think about the household and my recovery needs before the surgery actually happened. Chapter 9 goes into recovery planning in much more detail, but here are a few things that you might want to think about before the surgery happens.

ARRANGING POST-SURGICAL CARE

Before your surgery, take some time to think about who you would like to have as support during your immediate recovery. Tasks may be personal—showering, changing of surgical drains, and getting dressed. I decided that I wanted my husband to take care of these tasks for me. Perhaps you have another person who would be better suited for these other than your partner. If you live alone, think about who might be able to come in to help you. I highly advise you to have someone with you in the home for a few days after surgery. That way you will have support available if you need it.

ANTICIPATING PAIN MANAGEMENT

Pain management can present a challenge in recovery. When we are in too much pain, recovery is hampered because we are miserable. However, it is possible to develop dependencies to narcotic pain relievers in just a few days.[1] One of the new strategies that surgeons can use to ease pain, especially in mastectomy patients, is to administer a nerve block.[2] These are injections given in the pectoral area during the surgery that block pain for several days. A nerve block can reduce or eliminate the need for a narcotic pain reliever.

I recommend having a conversation with your surgeon during the pre-op appointment about strategies for pain management. It is important to keep the pain under control while avoiding dependency on opioid pain medications. To minimize this challenge at my home, I decided that I wanted my husband to help me monitor the medication doses. I wanted a record of what I took, but I didn't want to be the one writing everything down. I didn't want to risk becoming dependent on the medication, so I had him be responsible for the distribution. I was thankful that he would be the person notating when I had taken the medicine.

Another important thing is to figure out who will pick up the medications for you. We were able to get those filled at the hospital, but that option might not be available to you. If your surgery is in the afternoon, it might be a challenge to get those prescriptions filled before the pharmacy closes. Before your surgery, do a little research and figure out which pharmacies near your home or hospital stay open late into the evening. Doing so will avoid surgery-day scrambles trying to get to the pharmacy on time.

MANAGING TIME OFF WORK

Before your surgery, I would recommend that you work with your surgeon to get any paperwork signed and ready to go. Many companies have policies in place that require employees to give a medical rationale for taking more than a certain number of days off. Additionally, your company may have specific benefits available for more serious medical conditions.

Once you have made a surgical decision, I would recommend reaching out to your supervisor and your Human Resources department to see what time off is available. There may be a combination of paid and unpaid leave available.

As I was speaking with other ladies, they mentioned options that may be available if you don't have enough sick days to cover your recovery time. You could look into paid or unpaid family leave. Additionally, there may be options to take disability through your state. It may be possible to work out a flexible work arrangement with your boss. This could involve reduced hours each day, or perhaps a shorter work week. Working from home could also be an option as you begin to feel better.

How much time you might need to take off is dependent on what type of surgery you have, how your recovery is going, and whether or not you have complications.

I would recommend that you start by talking to your surgeon and seeing how long he thinks you might need to stay off work. When I talked to my surgeon, he thought my recovery time would be between two and three weeks. This information helped us fill out the family medical leave paperwork for Dave's job. His estimate was right on. I was feeling almost fully recovered after three weeks.

Since surgical recovery is so variable, I would recommend planning ahead for more time off than you may need. Being able to resume your job earlier than planned will be easier than asking for more time off. Overestimate your recovery time because unexpected challenges can come up.

WHERE TO LOOK IF YOU DON'T HAVE LIVE-IN SUPPORT

If you don't have live-in support during your surgical recovery, it may be necessary to reach out for extra help. Before your surgery, talk to your surgical team and see what type of social services might be available to help you take care of your recovery needs. There are companies that provide services specifically geared to people recovering from surgery alone.

I would start by talking to your doctor or nurse about your situation during your pre-op planning. It is possible that the doctor might recommend additional nights in the hospital for you so that you have the help you need. Perhaps your medical group can arrange for a home care nurse to come in and help you with specific tasks. There are also foundations and charities that offer help and support to cancer patients. I will put some of these links in the resource appendix.

I would recommend having a neighbor or friend available who is willing to be on call for you. This person could help you out by taking you to your medical appointments, running errands, or bringing in your mail.

If you are a part of a church or faith community, then I would reach out to them to see if there are ministries that can help you out. Our church offered to bring us dinners while I was in radiation. This was a big help to us, especially since Dave had returned to work.

One of the challenges that I faced during my recovery was accepting help. I am used to being capable of doing things for myself. But I needed others to come alongside me and help me through it. It is okay to ask for and accept help during this time.

OTHERS' JOURNEYS
PREPARING FOR SURGERY

As we prepare ourselves for surgery, we are also preparing our lives for change. Here are how some other women embraced support as they prepared for and recovered from surgery.

noelle "I have always used the phrase 'it takes a village,' and while I always valued those words and deep meaning, I now have a much more comprehensive understanding of its meaning. I, for one, allowed myself to be vulnerable and accepted help. This cancer road is hard enough, and no one should have to tough it out alone. Let your village help you in any aspect possible."[3]

nancy "I think what helped me was letting people be there for me. I had to surrender and accept that I needed help. Whether it was a meal train [or] people checking on me for emotional support. Also, my immediate family was a great part of preparing for surgery because it took away the stress of things that I would normally do. [Another thing that helped was] getting necessities like pillows, lotions, comfortable pj's, and clothes."[4]

joni "One of the ideas for pre-surgery especially if you have no one to help you the first few weeks, is to cook and freeze some heat-up meals. Also, plan to make an appointment to have your hair washed and blow-dried. If you can, hire a housekeeper or someone to come in to do some cleaning and laundry. I have a top that can hold your drains and has Velcro in place of buttons down the front; This top worked great while I had drains. Also, I found a sports bra (Fruit of the Loom) that used little hooks instead of a zipper that closed the front. [It was] much easier to use."[5]

MENTAL WELL-BEING
EMBRACING IMPERFECTION

I had so many things on my lists before surgery that I wasn't sure if it would all get done. Sometimes I would get spun up on how to prepare perfectly for recovery. I would get anxious and try to get everything done and forget to listen to my physical signals of exhaustion. It was in those moments of fatigue that I would yell at my kids or cry in my bed.

There is no way to prepare perfectly for surgery. I have given you some ideas in this chapter that might be helpful but are in no way comprehensive enough to cover everyone's unique needs.

I encourage you to embrace imperfection during this time. Whatever doesn't get done before surgery will either stay undone until you can get to it later, or someone else will do it.

EMOTIONAL WELL-BEING

FEAR OF THE UNKNOWN

Heading into surgery is an emotional time. I had a lot of fear going into surgery day. I had never been under general anesthesia, and the thought of it terrified me. I didn't know if I was going to wake up. I was scared about how I would recover. I didn't know what my breasts would look like when the cancer was removed. There were so many unknowns and I found that the more I focused on them, the more emotional I became.

There were also many hoops to jump through. I had phone calls to make and appointments to attend. I got frustrated because all those things to do took away from my ability to be home with my kids and enjoy them before my surgery.

Some of the strategies that I tried to use when I was feeling emotional during this time included:

- Deep breathing
- Meditation
- Visualizing myself relaxing on a tropical beach
- Prayer
- Writing Bible verses of comfort in my journal
- Walking outside
- Playing fun games on my phone or tablet
- Talking with my close friends and family
- Making small talk with the medical professionals
- Writing my feelings down
- Crying (not a strategy, but it was helpful!)
- Laughing with my family

Emotions can be all over the place before surgery. I'm surprised that I got any sleep at all the night before my lumpectomy. I remember packing the bag and checking my list right before I headed to bed. I kept checking to see if there was anything left to do. It was all done. The only thing left to do was to show up on time in the morning. I set the alarm for 4 a.m., turned the lights out, and snuggled up against Dave for the night.

8

SURGERY DAY
facing the unknown

THE RHYTHMIC BEEPING OF my alarm interrupted my fitful dreams. Bleary-eyed, I reached for my phone and turned on the lights. My surgery wasn't until the afternoon, but if I wanted to eat anything, I needed to finish my breakfast before 5 a.m. There was no way I was going to face my day without something to eat and a cup of coffee!

In this chapter, I'll share the details of my surgery day and also some things that I learned along the way. I discovered that even though I had made lots of lists in preparation, there were things I hadn't anticipated. I faced the unknown with as much preparation as I could. This was the day we had been waiting for.

MY JOURNEY
COMPLICATED EMOTIONS

I remember feeling a tumultuous mix of emotions that morning. I was anxious and worried, but also grateful that the day had finally arrived. My planner for the day had no to-dos, only the words "Surgery Day" at the top. Underneath was a Bible verse I had written out in the morning:

Psalm 73: 23-26 (World English Version)

Nevertheless, I am continually with you.
You have held my right hand.
You will guide me with your counsel,
and afterward receive me to glory.
Whom do I have in heaven?
There is no one on earth whom
I desire besides you.
My flesh and my heart fails,
but God is the strength of my
heart and my portion forever.

I was headed into a day of unknowns, and these words provided me the encouragement that I was longing for.

Before Dave and I left for the hospital at 8:30, I had him take pictures of me and the kids. I had considered writing letters to my kids before the surgery in case something happened to me, but I never followed through on that idea. Pictures would have to do. As we smiled for the camera, fleeting thoughts of the worst-case scenarios flooded through my brain. The hugs lasted longer than usual and then we were off. There was a schedule to keep.

My lumpectomy procedure only took a few hours, but the procedures before and the recovery from anesthesia afterward made for a long day.

LOCALIZATION BEFORE SURGERY

The first step in my day was to have a localization procedure done in the radiology department. This was essential because my DCIS was not visible to the naked eye. The localization provided a way for the surgeon to know exactly where the DCIS was during the lumpectomy.

There are a few different ways that localization can be done. Some surgeons will do this a few days before by injecting a wireless marker into the precise location to be removed. This wire-free localization procedure is similar to that of a biopsy.[1]

My surgeon used a traditional method of wire localization. This type of localization used a thin wire to mark the location of the area to be removed.[2] I needed to arrive a few hours before surgery to get this procedure done. In my case, the procedure was done by a radiologist in the women's imaging center across the street from the hospital.

Dave dropped me off at the women's center so that he could find a place to park. I walked into the office as if it was a regular appointment. "I'm here to check in for my localization," I said to the receptionists. I had no idea what was ahead of me, but this was the first step.

I sat down by myself in the waiting room feeling unsure and fearful. Nothing was familiar to me. My chest tightened, and my breathing became shallow. I was regretting that I'd told Dave I would be okay by myself. I breathed a sigh of relief when I saw him come through the door. His presence calmed me down in the few moments we were able to sit together.

"Mrs. Douglas?" called the nurse. It was my turn, and my heart was pounding. I followed the nurse through the doors, feeling anxious and worried. The first stop was the changing room. I left my belongings in a locker and put on the pink radiology robe.

The nurse reminded me that I would have two wires placed. One would mark the DCIS to be removed and the other would mark the benign fibroadenoma. The radiologist would use two different imaging techniques to guide the wire placement.

The first wire to be placed was the one for the fibroadenoma. The ultrasound room was dimly lit and had a floral mural painted on the wall. I laid down on the table and the tech positioned me so that I was lying comfortably on my back with my left breast uncovered. My imaging was visible on the back wall for reference. The tech used the ultrasound to find the correct area. The radiologist came in, and then moved the wand to the underside of my left breast. Confused, I looked up at him and exclaimed, "What are you doing? That is the wrong place!"

He responded, "Well, that's what I see on the imaging."

I had multiple benign lesions in the left breast, and he was going to place the wire in the wrong fibroadenoma. The one my surgeon planned to remove was on the top of my left breast. Remember when I said that it is important to know exactly where the lumps are? This is why! If I hadn't known, the wrong finding would be removed.

The radiologist wasn't about to take my word for it. My calm demeanor covered up my internal anger and frustration. I was the patient, and I knew what I was talking about. Looking back, I can see that he was being thorough and detailed, but at the time I was really frustrated. I had been up since 4 a.m., and my stomach was growling.

I wanted this day to be over with and didn't want any more delays.

The radiologist had my surgeon paged. He said, "I don't know if I'm going to be able to get hold of him if he is in surgery. I will be back when I get confirmation." He left the room to go do other procedures, leaving me lying on the table in the ultrasound room staring at the mural and wondering how long I would wait. I was terrified that this communication mishap would derail my surgery. Thankfully, the ultrasound tech stayed with me for the half an hour it took to get the answer. If I had been left alone in the room, I think I would have worked myself into even more of a panic. The small talk we made was calming and distracting. Her demeanor was reassuring and caring.

After what seemed like forever, the radiologist returned with the confirmation he needed. The surgeon told him exactly which fibroadenoma to mark: the one I had told him about. He was all business as he began. Clearly, the delay didn't seem to have bothered him at all. Perhaps things like this happened frequently. I tried to breathe deeply and let my frustration go now that the procedure was beginning. I didn't want to pass out as I had for my mammogram-guided biopsy, so I closed my eyes and focused on my breathing.

The radiologist numbed me using a local anesthetic. I felt the pinch, the burn, and then the cold feeling as my breast became numb. Once I was numb, he was ready to insert the thin and flexible wire. He pressed it into my skin and attempted to maneuver it into the fibroadenoma. The mass was slippery and kept moving around. Eventually, he used the ultrasound wand to keep the lump in one place and used his other hand to push the wire through the mass. I squeezed my eyes shut and prayed that I wouldn't black out.

At this point, I felt like a fish on a hook. I was hungry, cranky, and had a wire sticking out of me—and there was one more localization to go. So far, I was not enjoying surgery day.

Next, I needed to move to the mammogram room to have my DCIS localized. Someone else was in there so I needed to wait again. As I sat in the uncomfortable chair, I felt vulnerable and alone. I tried not to think about the wire that was poking out of my left breast. Thankfully, it had been taped down with some gauze.

When it was finally my turn, I made sure to tell the techs that I had passed out during my mammogram-guided biopsy. I was already feeling quite weak because of the emotional frustration and the fasting. I was concerned that I would need to stand up for this procedure, but thankfully there was a chair ready.

One of the techs in the room was in charge of keeping me talking and distracted. The other tech was in charge of the computer and positioning. I was busy and occupied talking about my family while the medical procedure continued.

First, they placed me in compression and gave me a mammogram. The mammogram was used to determine the location of the biopsy clip. Then I was numbed again. The wire was inserted into the correct area while I was still under compression. This process went much faster because the wire hooked right into the biopsy clip.

Once I was finished, they took more mammograms of the wires. I was wrapped up so that the wires weren't sticking straight out, and then I could get dressed. I was handed the mammogram films to take with me to the hospital. I had arrived around 10 a.m. at the women's center for the localization process and it was now nearly 12:30. I was really hungry and concerned I would be late to my own surgery.

I was so happy to see my husband and his friend Dale waiting for me in the room. Tears flooded my eyes as I hugged both of them. The last time I had seen Dale was at the funeral for his wife, Dora. She had passed away from metastatic breast cancer a year or so before my diagnosis. I was grateful Dave would have Dale with him as I headed into surgery.

HOSPITAL CHECK-IN: ASK FOR A WHEELCHAIR!

The hospital provided a van for Dave and me to go across the street for check in. This was before COVID-19 restrictions, so Dave was able to come with me until they took me to the surgery room. Lots of people were waiting around in the lobby, and there was a line to get through the check-in process. I felt self-conscious and wondered if everyone could see the wires underneath my shirt.

I was woozy and nervous about the surgery, especially since I was in an unfamiliar hospital. Nothing felt comforting or safe. There weren't a lot of places to sit, so Dave found me a chair and then waited in the hallway. Finally, a clerk was available so that we could get the check-in completed. I was assigned a number that Dave would be able to use to track the progress of my surgery. Viewable on the screens in the waiting area, the graphic used color-coded symbols to represent where I was in the process.

The next step was to get me to the correct floor. The hospital was under construction, and there was a lot of walking to do. I soon wished I had asked for a wheelchair.

We arrived at the surgery floor and then were directed to yet another waiting room. There were a few other people there who were also waiting for their loved ones. Between the conversations about gory surgical details and the loud television, I found it difficult to stay calm. The waiting room was so small that there was no way to escape and have a private moment of peace with Dave.

FINALLY GETTING A ROOM

Finally, a room opened up on my floor so that I could get checked in. I was relieved to be able to leave that waiting room and the disturbing conversations. The nurse handed me a packet of warm wipes and walked us into a private hospital room.

I had specific wiping and cleaning procedures to go through to minimize the risk of bacterial infection. Every hospital has a different procedure. I have spoken with some patients who need to use a special surgical soap in the shower for several days before surgery. If that is the case, your surgeon or nurse should call you to clarify.

I got clean and then got under the blankets and waited for the nurse to come in. As I warmed up on the bed, I felt a peace and calm come over me. After all the biopsies, imaging, and blood tests, the surgery was less than an hour away. So much planning and preparing had gone into this moment. I was in the surgical bed, and soon the cancer would be out of me.

The nurse came in and asked me numerous questions about my medical history. She took copious notes and then went over my aftercare instructions. It was going to be important for Dave to watch me carefully after surgery to reduce my risk of falling.

Once she had the answers she needed, she placed the IV and collected my belongings in a bag, which would be waiting in the recovery room.

As I was chatting with the nurse, I shared that I was nervous about going under anesthesia. She recommended that I think happy thoughts as I was being sedated and explained that those emotions would be the ones I'd wake up with. Since I had never been under anesthesia before, I had no idea if she was right. It seemed like a good suggestion, so I decided to try it out.

TIME FOR SURGERY

A phone call came into the nurse's station. It was my surgeon calling to see if I was ready. It was 2:15, and he was waiting. The orderlies came into my room, unlocked the wheels on my bed, and pushed me out the door. Dave could walk with me until the doors to the surgical area, and then it was time to say goodbye. That was a hard goodbye to say. We kissed, and then they pushed me through the doors.

In this unfamiliar hospital, I felt like just another number in their system. Then I heard my surgeon's voice as he chatted with the other doctors, and I felt my stress level go down. He hadn't seen me come into the hallway yet, but hearing his familiar voice made me feel better. Once he noticed I was there, he came over, touched my arm and asked, "How are you doing?"

"I'm nervous," I told him.

Then the anesthesiologist came over. All I remember is that she said that she didn't like to count down for her patients. I would have the mask over me, and then I would fall asleep.

They wheeled me into the cold operating room. I saw my name along with my drug and adhesive allergies written on the white board. I could see the mammogram films from the localization process in the light table next to the whiteboard. There were so many people in the room! I was surprised that there would be so many people involved in my care who I would likely never meet again. Then I was moved to the table. One of the nurses introduced herself. She said her job would be to monitor my vital signs throughout the procedure and make sure I was okay. That was reassuring.

The last thing I remember after moving to the table was a mask being put on my face. I thought about my family and breathed deeply.

WAKING UP

When I woke up, I looked around and realized I was in a different room. I turned to my left and asked the nurse, "Is it over?"

"Yes," she said and smiled.

I burst into joyful tears. I couldn't believe it. I had made it. I started shivering a bit, and she injected some Demerol into my IV. I immediately felt calm and at peace.

Relief and happiness flooded through me. I guess the nurse was right. I was thinking happy thoughts about my family, and then I woke up feeling joyful.

I looked around for my surgeon, but he wasn't there anymore. I found out later that after my lumpectomy was finished, he met with Dave to tell him how the surgery had gone and to give aftercare instructions. It was so surreal to be in the operating room one moment and recovery the next.

"How did it go?" I asked the nurse.

"Everything went well," she told me.

Then two orderlies came to move me back down to a private room to recover.

I was in the room for just a little while when I heard Dave's voice in the hallway as he was working out some logistics with the nurses about my prescriptions. I was so excited to see him that I wanted to jump out of bed, but I think I was still hooked up to an IV.

He came in and gave me a big, gentle hug. I could see the look of relief in his eyes. The nurses had me get up and walk around a little bit, explaining that I needed to be able to walk and use the restroom before they would release me to go home. They also were monitoring my pulse and blood pressure.

After I used the restroom, the nurses were comfortable letting me get ready to go home. It was after 5:30 and I was thrilled to get out of the hospital and home to my safe, cozy bed. We needed to wait until the pain medication arrived from the pharmacy, and then I could get dressed. I had no idea what I would look like once I opened the hospital gown. I remember feeling uncomfortable as I slid the gown off and looked down at my chest. There was not much to see since my breasts were wrapped up tightly, mummy-style. My surgeon used this instead of tape because I'm allergic to adhesives. The cloth bandage would need to stay in place until I had an appointment with him the following week. Unfortunately, it meant I would need to go over a week without a traditional shower.

Surprisingly, I had woken up without surgical drains. I'll discuss these more in detail in the next chapter, because they are a common component of surgical recovery. I wanted to race to get dressed and leave, but I was still a bit woozy from all the anesthesia and exhausted from the long day. Slow was the appropriate pace to make sure I didn't forget anything, hurt myself, or fall before I'd even gotten home.

This time, they wheeled me through the halls and out the doors of the hospital. Dave asked, "Do you feel up to walking to the car? I'm not too far away, and I think it might be hard to get back here with all the construction."

"Sure, as long as we go slow," I replied. I got up carefully, and we walked gingerly, arm and arm, to the car. I was thrilled to be heading home after a long and emotional day.

THE FLOW OF SURGERY DAY

Surgery day is a unique one because it flows at the pace of the hospital, not at our pace. We can want the day to be over, but it won't be until the pre-determined flow has finished. Time slows for us as we head into the surgery, but then there are hours missing from our memory when we wake up. Every hospital has its own flow, and we join it briefly, as patients, and then head home, while the flow continues without us.

BEFORE SURGERY

I was surprised at how much needed to be done before the surgery could take place. In my case, it was a localization procedure and a lengthy check-in process. Your day may flow differently than mine because of how your hospital arranges for surgeries.

Hospital Check-in/Admission. Even if your surgery is planned as an outpatient procedure, you will likely need to go through the standard hospital admission process. This usually involves signing forms and answering lots of questions. This is likely when you'll get a hospital wristband.

Localizing. If your surgeon uses a wire to localize before the surgery, this placement will happen on the day of surgery. In my case, it was done before my hospital check-in, but I've also heard of women who have this procedure done after they are admitted to the hospital. If your surgeon uses a wire-free localizing device, this procedure might be done on a different day.

Sentinel Lymph Node Biopsy. This is a procedure done to see if the cancer has spread to the lymph nodes. A blue dye and/or a radioactive substance is injected near the tumor. This enables the surgeon to identify the lymph node closest to the tumor, known as the sentinel node, and remove it during surgery. This might be done on the day before your surgery, if you're having a morning surgery, or on the day of the surgery. I have learned from other survivors that your urine might be blue in the few days after your surgery, so don't be surprised if that happens.

Getting Settled and Changed. Once you have finished the check-in process, it is time to get into the hospital gown. Every hospital has a slightly different procedure for this, but hopefully you'll get a nice warm blanket when you get in the hospital bed.

Nursing Conversations and IV Placement. Once you're changed and tucked into the hospital bed, it is time for the conversations with your pre-surgical nursing team. They have a list of questions and tests to go over with you and will place the IV for your surgery. One of the questions I got asked multiple times during surgery day was "When was the last time I had anything to eat or drink?" So, make sure to keep track of that so you can answer it, over and over!

SURGERY TIME

At some point, all of the pre-surgery tasks will be completed, and the surgical team takes over. If your partner has been able to be with you during the pre-surgery time, this is likely when you'll say goodbye to him/her. During the surgery, the hospital team will have the ability to communicate progress with your partner.

Moving to the Surgery Department. You'll be moved, in a hospital bed, to the surgery department once everyone is ready for you. I took some of my belongings with me, like my glasses and my post-surgery bra, and some of them were stored for me during surgery.

Anesthesiology. Before you are administered the general anesthesia, you'll have the opportunity to talk with the anesthesiologist. She will likely ask you questions about any previous experiences you had with general anesthesia and will ask about the last time you ate or drank.

Surgical Nursing Team. There will be a dedicated nursing team for your surgery, and you might meet them briefly before the surgery.

Surgeon. In my case, the only time I talked to my surgeon was just before surgery. He confirmed the surgery and made sure that any questions I had before the procedure were answered. He also checked to confirm the locations of the areas to be removed and looked at the wires.

Operating Room. Depending on the flow of your hospital, you might be awake as you transition to the operating room table, or you may already be under anesthesia. It is a bright and busy room, and I was surprised at how many people were involved in my surgery.

POST-SURGERY

Once the surgery is complete, you'll be moved into the recovery area and monitored for any complications. It's startling to wake up in a different place with a different team around you. I remember feeling relieved it was over and ready to get out of the hospital.

> **Recovery Area.** I was surprised to wake up and be in a recovery area with other patients. The nursing team was keeping a close eye on us, checking on our vitals consistently. Depending on your hospital, you might be released directly from the recovery area, or you might be moved back to a hospital room.

> **Hospital Release.** I was ready to leave as soon as I opened my eyes after surgery, but that wasn't how things worked. In order for the hospital to clear you for release, you'll need to be monitored for a certain period of time and demonstrate that you can go home safely. The medical team needs to clear you for release, and then you can begin the transition home. The IV will be removed, and you'll be able to change into your clothes. If the medical team determines that it will be better for you to stay in the hospital, then this might be the next day. Some surgeries, such as flap reconstruction, are done as in-patient procedures and you'll be staying in the hospital for a time to be monitored for any complications.

There are so many aspects of surgery day that are out of our immediate control. There was a culture, a flow, and a way the hospital did things. My surgeon was the only recognizable face on my medical team that day. As the timing proceeded at their pace, not mine, I was reminded just why we are called patients.

OTHERS' JOURNEYS
UNEXPECTED CHALLENGES DURING & AFTER SURGERY

It is uncomfortable to think about what challenges might arise during or after surgery. But it is possible to experience them. As much as we plan and prepare, we cannot control all the aspects of what happens in the operating room or during our recovery.

sandy "I had my lumpectomy on December 4, 2019, and everything went well, she got clear margins, so then I was scheduled for reconstructive surgery on December 11, 2019. I was told that he (the plastic surgeon) would either remove my large implants that day or replace them with smaller implants when he did the reconstruction. I woke up after surgery to find out that he did neither. He left my original implants in. When I asked why, he said that he didn't think I would be happy with no implants and the smaller implants that he ordered for me were smaller in size, but they were high profile, and my old implants were low profile, so he thought it would be best to leave the original implants in. I was so upset that day. It was very frustrating that a plastic surgeon would make a decision like that."[3]

noelle Ended up needing a second surgery. "After three and a half weeks, my last drain was finally removed. Praise be to God. I couldn't wait to shower like a normal human being. Within 12 hours of the last drain being pulled, my left breast became very red and hot. Through the evening I developed a high fever and had the chills. Turns out, I developed an infection and had to be admitted back into the hospital. It was determined that I had to go back into surgery to remove the implant, clean out the entire left side, and place a new implant, and unfortunately new drains were also placed. While I hated that I had a second surgery, my recovery from this one went much smoother, which told me that I had issues from the get-go. I was placed on a home IV to continue to fight the infection for 14 days. I have not had any issues since. The entire process was very emotional for me."[4]

janelle Initially had a lumpectomy, then had a mastectomy. "My surgery decision was one of the hardest decisions I've ever made in my life. I spent several weeks weighing the pros and cons and getting second and third opinions from surgeons. It was hard because both options were bad in my mind. I ultimately chose to have a lumpectomy with radiation over a mastectomy, out of pure fear of the surgery and reconstruction. A week after my lumpectomy, the surgeon called to tell me the margins were not clear and they found more cancer in what was thought was a non-cancer breast. The decision to have a double mastectomy then became so easy. I learned a hard lesson that day: some things are not up to me."[5]

MENTAL WELL-BEING
EXPECTING THE UNEXPECTED ON SURGERY DAY

It isn't possible for us to predict all of the challenges we may face, or the complications that might arise during surgery. A flexible mindset can help us better manage these challenges as they happen.

I thought that I was done with delays and surprises when I arrived at the women's center for my localization procedure. I was not expecting that the localization would be delayed because the radiologist and the surgeon didn't communicate well enough about the exact location of my fibroadenoma.

Stepping back now, I can see that the delay was out of caution. The radiologist wanted to make sure he did the best job possible so that my surgery would be successful. But his reluctance to listen to me provoked anxiety, frustration, and the feeling of powerlessness. I was awake, and this problem was happening. What if something like that happened when I was under anesthesia? I wouldn't be able to advocate for myself.

If I ever head back into another surgery, I will go into it with a different mindset. I will be more open and flexible, knowing that the unexpected might happen. If I'm able to advocate for myself in a medical situation, I will. However, if I'm under anesthesia then I will need to trust that my surgeon, or my husband, will make the necessary medical decisions at the time.

EMOTIONAL WELL-BEING
VOICING OUR FEARS & CONCERNS

One of the ways that I tried to support my emotional well-being during treatment was to be vocal and open about my fears and concerns. I discovered that talking about my emotions enabled me to get support in new ways both before and during the procedures.

One of my biggest fears was about going under anesthesia for the first time. I had talked to my friends and family, and they were all encouraging. A family member told me that general anesthesia was like taking a great nap. I valued their perspectives, but I still was worried.

I decided that I would be very up front with my medical team about my fears. Before my surgery, I clarified with my surgeon which type of anesthesia he would be using during the procedure. Given my previous experiences with the biopsies, I hoped I didn't need to be awake during the actual surgery. After he told me it would be under general anesthesia, I was relieved, but also terrified of a new experience.

On surgery day, I talked to the admitting nurse about how worried I was about undergoing general anesthesia. I asked her how they determined if I was able to go home after waking up. In addition, I made sure to share my fears and concerns with the anesthesiology team before I went under.

I discovered that voicing my fears and concerns allowed me to acknowledge my feelings. Conversely, these conversations with the medical providers helped them understand my emotional state. Additionally, I felt empowered and calmer after speaking with them.

A JOYFUL REUNION AT HOME

I couldn't believe surgery was over. I was still giddy from the anesthesia. The forty-five-minute ride home went by in a blur. I made a few celebratory calls to family then I relaxed for the rest of the ride.

We got home and Dave helped me get settled on the couch. By this time, it was 7:30 and we were ready for a little food and an early bedtime. It had been a long day for all of us. I ate a little something, and then we were ready for the kids to walk home from Scott and Judee's house. They bounded in, holding their project from the day. It was a bright pink pumpkin with a ribbon carved in it. In all the hustle and bustle of getting ready for surgery, we hadn't carved pumpkins together. What an amazing and touching project they had worked on all day.

I hugged the kids, gently, with a heart full of joy and gratitude. After sharing how my day went, and listening to their stories from the day, I was ready to get to bed. It was almost 10, and I was exhausted. Dave guided me upstairs and helped me get into my pajamas. That night, I was able to sleep more soundly than I had in months. The anxiety and worry were gone. Surgery was done. Now it was time to switch gears towards recovery.

PART II

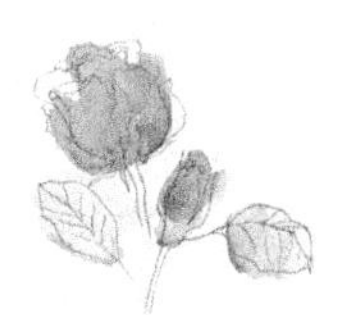

Post-Surgery

ADDITIONAL
TREATMENT
DECISIONS
& RECOVERY

9 SOFT LANDING
optimizing for early recovery

THE BEAMS OF LIGHT streaming through the shutters shocked me out of my deep sleep. I always woke up before the sunrise. What was going on? The day before, I'd woken up with worry and anxiety. I examined my fuzzy morning brain for those emotions. They were gone. For the first time in months, I had slept soundly. I had made it through the surgery and the cancer was out. The anxiety and worry had melted away overnight. It was time to begin a new step in this journey.

Recovery from breast cancer surgery can be a confusing swirl. I remember feeling peace and joy that the surgery was finished but also frustrated that I still had activity restrictions. By anticipating and preparing for this post-surgical swirl, we can optimize our homes and lives for the recovery process.

MY JOURNEY
CHALLENGES IN DELEGATING

It was hard for me to let go of my normal responsibilities. I wanted to jump in and take over because it was "my job." One of the most memorable lessons that I learned during this recovery period was that other people were just as capable of managing the home as I was. When I began to realize this, it was a real challenge to my self-worth. I had been managing the home for years and took a lot of pride in doing it. I had defined the ways we did things in the home. Now, Dave and the boys were doing it their way. We had a few bumps in the road as they took over the home management.

DAY 1: THE COFFEE DEBACLE

After we woke up on the first day after surgery, Dave helped me get downstairs to the couch. I was looking forward to a lovely hot cup of coffee. Dave walked over to the coffeemaker, picked up the pot, and then grimaced. There were grounds all over the place and dried coffee all over the black countertop. The pot hadn't been set in the machine just right and the coffee had overflowed and made a huge mess.

I tried to jump up and help, and he quickly told me to stay put. He salvaged a cup for me and then set to work cleaning. As I sat there, drinking my coffee, he went into cleaning mode. He was going to take care of that entire mess and make sure that it never happened again. Unfortunately, in the process of cleaning it, the electronics in the coffeemaker got damaged.

This recovery was not getting off to a good start. It was the first day, and the coffee pot was going to the trash. I had a difficult choice to make. I could judge him and tell him the right way to solve the problem, or I could sit back and let him engineer a solution.

We had a spare coffee pot that we used for a while, but Dave was convinced there was a better way to brew coffee. He did extensive research and found out the correct number of grams needed for each pot. Then he found a coffee pot that would get the water to the exact right temperature to brew the "golden cup." When he was finally done architecting the solution, we had a new coffee pot, hooked up to a smart plug, that brews the best coffee I have ever had.

I smile every time I pour myself a cup of coffee now. Dave reinvented our morning coffee, for the better. What other changes might be possible if I let go of the home-making reins just a bit?

CHILDREN

This was a hard time for our kids. It was the first time I had been so unavailable to them. They were dealing with challenging emotions, brand-new daily routines without me, increased chores, and fears that I might die. We discovered that when they could help me out, they were able to participate and assist tangibly in my recovery. They could also see me getting better.

The boys were excellent "runners" when I needed things. I would send a text message to the family when I was hungry or thirsty. A few minutes later, a boy would knock on the door and bring me the snack. They would take down my dishes and warm up my heating pad. Dave had the boys jumping to it every time.

At first, I felt guilty asking for so much help from them. They didn't ask for their mom to get cancer, and now they had a lot more work than they were used to. Looking back, I see it differently. This recovery offered them a unique opportunity to participate actively in my healing process. I watched them learn how to demonstrate care and love to me in a new and constructive way. Over the years, I had done many things for them when they couldn't, and now it was their chance to help me out.

Another chore the boys did regularly during my recovery was walking our rambunctious beagles. This was usually something that Dave and I did together, but I wasn't allowed to walk long distances for a few weeks. Every evening, they would leash up the beagles and take them around the neighborhood. This was a precious time because they could talk about how they were really doing, without my hearing. While I don't know exactly what they talked about, I did hear later that there was a lot of venting during those dog walks.

It's possible that your children might be struggling during your cancer treatment. If the strong emotions are getting overwhelming for you and your partner, consider seeking professional support. This will allow your children to talk about their emotions in a more neutral environment.

FAMILY & FRIENDS

My family and friends were a big support during my treatment and recovery. They would call, text, or visit to brighten my day. Before my surgery, I would walk once a week with Rebekah. That wasn't an option after my surgery, but she would visit and bring me a mocha. I had other friends drop by and just spend time talking to me.

Another way that my friends were able to help was by running errands. Maybe it was picking up coffee or dropping something off at the post office. When someone offered to help, I tried to think of something simple they could do that would take something off of Dave's plate. This helped him focus on keeping the household running during my initial recovery.

Whether it was phone calls from family who didn't live nearby, visits that cheered me up, flowers that brightened my room, or text messages from my extended support network, I discovered that help and support was all around me.

Gradually, I began to feel better about letting go of my usual responsibilities. There were others who could take care of these things for me. It was a big emotional step to let go of the guilt. I didn't have to do all the homemaking tasks to be worthwhile. Accepting help wasn't easy, but that help was a tangible expression of the love surrounding us during my cancer journey.

SETTING UP THE HOME FOR THE BEST RECOVERY POSSIBLE

Even if everything goes smoothly, you will need time to recover from surgery. It helps to plan ahead about what you will need to have a stress-free recovery. Below are a few things I thought about when planning for this time.

RECOVERY SPACE

One of the first things that I thought about was where I wanted my primary recovery space to be. Initially, I thought that the best place was downstairs on the couch. I would be available to help out as needed, and it would be easy for the family to bring me things. Dave shot this idea down. I remember him looking at me and saying, "You need to have your own space to recover. I don't want you to get pulled into the school. You don't need that stress when you're trying to heal."

I hadn't really spent a lot of time thinking about how stressful my daily routine was, but he was right. My everyday work all happened downstairs. The school room was right next to the couch. The kids were used to asking me for help when they had a challenging lesson. The kitchen and laundry room were just a few steps away. Would I really be able to focus on my recovery when I was in my home office?

After much discussion, we decided that the best place for me to recover would be in my bedroom. This would keep me physically out of the homeschool area. If I wasn't there, they couldn't ask me questions. In my room, I could sleep and rest whenever I wanted to. I could have phone calls and visitors without disrupting the homeschool environment. It ended up being an ideal space for me to recover.

As you prepare for surgery, think about where you would like to do your initial recovery. Ideally, you will have a comfortable space where you can sit up for a while, and then relax for a nap. It should be near a bathroom and have a place for you to put comfort items like a water bottle, snacks, things to do, and chargers for your electronic devices. I have spoken to women who have recovered in their rooms, like I did. Others had a recliner or an adjustable mattress. Recliners specifically designed for surgical recovery can be rented from medical supply companies.

The first few weeks, I spent a lot of time in my bed recuperating. I was able to enjoy the view outside and have separation from the homeschool. Being away enabled me to prioritize my physical, mental, and emotional recovery. I had time to think about what I had been through and process some of the feelings that came up.

My surgeon estimated that my recovery from the lumpectomy would be between two to three weeks. Recovery from a mastectomy can be longer, usually anywhere from four to eight weeks. The timeframe for returning to work may vary based on your job duties, surgical choices, and post-surgery treatment choices. I recommend getting an estimate from your surgeon as to anticipated recovery time and then revise as needed.

PRIMARY CAREGIVER

I wanted Dave to be my primary caregiver. I needed help with dressing and showering for a few weeks, and I wasn't comfortable with anyone else doing those jobs. For a week after surgery, the only way I could get clean was with a sponge bath.

It isn't necessary to have your partner be your primary caregiver. I have spoken with women who have had their moms or adult children come and help them. During my biopsy phase, my mom helped wrap my breasts up in a bandage so that I didn't bleed in the bed at night. I'm glad she was there to help me, because wrapping the bandage myself was nearly impossible.

As I mentioned before, I didn't have surgical drains placed after my lumpectomy. Drains are standard after a mastectomy and will need to be drained and managed for several weeks. It will be quite helpful to have your caregiver perform that task for you.

Also, I recommend having your caregiver keep track of your medication doses. There may be several prescriptions to manage, and it is important to take the right amount of medicine. Dave kept track of the medicine and wrote down when I took each dose. I'm glad that I didn't need to think about that during my recovery. I was worried about becoming dependent on pain meds, but I knew that being in pain would make my recovery more challenging. Asking Dave for help with monitoring my medications lowered my stress and helped me feel comfortable that I was taking the right amount of pain medicine.

HOUSEHOLD HELP

Another thing to consider is who will be managing the rest of the house while you recover. We had some unique issues to address because we are a virtual schooling family. It was important to me was that the kids didn't fall behind in their classes. My older son, Ken, was taking a difficult course load as a junior in high school and my younger son, Dan, had just started high school. Dan was learning how to manage multiple teachers and a much more difficult school day.

Dave took time off through the family leave program in order to run the homeschool while I was recovering. This family leave was arranged through his work and was a combination of our state benefits for paid family leave and additional benefits he had through work.

At some point during his time as a substitute homemaker and learning coach, he came up to the bedroom to fold some clothes. He looked at me and said, "It is so strange: if I'm downstairs, the boys do fine at school. But, if I leave, there's trouble." I smiled at him. He was figuring out what my days were like!

I ended up delegating all of my homemaking and schooling tasks to Dave for three weeks. He took over the cooking, the laundry, and the dog walking. It was a crash course for him in household management.

FOOD—WE NEEDED LOTS OF IT!

We have two teenage boys who are hungry all the time. At first, Dave would go to the grocery store to do the shopping. But this meant that he wasn't home to supervise the homeschooling. We needed to come up with a better strategy.

Eventually, we decided to have the groceries delivered and planned a few nights a week of takeout. This strategy helped him have less to manage throughout the day. We also had friends and our church family offer to bring us meals. That was another huge blessing to our family. Initially, I felt uncomfortable saying yes to the meals. Dave was home and able to prepare food, but he was also managing the homeschool and caring for me. Having the meals taken care of for the night was a relief. I quickly learned to say yes any time someone offered to bring us dinner!

I tried to stock up on the household staples before surgery. I thought about the snacks I would want to eat and the cleaning supplies we needed. I didn't want us running out of laundry detergent the first day of recovery.

DO HOUSECLEANING & LAUNDRY BEFORE SURGERY

As I mentioned in the previous chapter, I would highly recommend cleaning the house and doing your laundry, if those are a part of your routines, *before* your surgery. These are physically demanding chores and you won't be able to do them during your recovery. I made sure to change my sheets right before surgery because that was a task that required lots of reaching, and I knew I wouldn't be able to do it.

I recommend hiring help for cleaning if you aren't able to do it yourself. During my research, I discovered a charity called *Cleaning for a Reason* that will provide free, once-a-month cleaning for four months for cancer patients in the United States and Canada. I have included a link in the resource guide. This task could also be something a friend might be willing to do for you. I really enjoyed having a clean home to recover in.

Before my surgery, my mom searched the house high and low for every single piece of laundry she could do. She got it all clean, folded, and put away. It was such a huge help to have that done before my surgery. I remember feeling bad that she was visiting and doing "my job." What I didn't realize at the time was that her help was therapeutic for her. She couldn't take away the cancer, but she could do my laundry for me.

PET CARE

Think about who will be responsible for the dog walking, noise patrol, and poop pick up after your surgery. These tasks will be difficult for you to manage during the first few weeks. We had our dogs stay with the house sitter for a few days after my surgery. After that, Dave and the boys would walk them.

If you have cats, think about who will be able to empty the cat litter. This might be a difficult physical task to handle, and if you are undergoing chemotherapy, you won't be allowed to do so. While you are undergoing chemo, your immune system will be compromised. Since dirty cat litter carries a risk of toxoplasmosis, it is advised that you avoid changing the litter yourself during treatment. I recommend checking with your oncologist about any pet care tasks you do regularly and ensure that they are safe for you to do during chemo.

RELOCATING REGULARLY USED ITEMS TO LOWER SHELVES

It is common to have movement restrictions for your arms, especially after a mastectomy. The general recommendation is to not lift or reach for things that are above your shoulders. So, if you have regularly used items that live on the top shelf of your cabinets or closets, I recommend moving them to lower shelves so it is easier for you to reach. During my recovery, I made sure to hang the shirts I wanted to wear on a lower rod in my closet so I wasn't reaching for them and disturbing my stitches.

PRACTICAL ITEMS FOR THE FIRST FEW DAYS OF RECOVERY

I had several things that were helpful for me during the first few days. I'll include links to some of my favorite ones in the resource appendix for easy purchasing:

Soft, Button-Up Pajamas. The buttons made these easy to get on and off. I felt comfortable enough in these pajamas that I would wear them when I had visitors.

Front-Close Sports Bras. You will not be pulling things over your head during your early recovery. There are a few different ways that front-close bras can be made. My favorite ones were made of a soft cotton and had hook-and-eye closures. These didn't irritate me the way zippers or Velcro did.

Clothing Items for Drain Management. There are various specialty items designed to make living with surgical drains a little easier. These can range from pouches to robes with built-in pockets, or shirts with interior drain pockets. Special clothing isn't a necessity since the drains can be attached to your existing items with safety pins.

Water Bottle. I really liked drinking cold water, so I had a water bottle that was made of double walled stainless steel. It would keep my water ice cold for hours. It also had a good seal, so if I knocked it over it wouldn't get all over my electronics.

Wedge Pillow. I would not have been able to sleep without this pillow. I could use it for sleeping by placing it on its low setting. When I was ready to sit up in bed and read, I would turn it to the tall setting and lean against it. The one I chose was made of foam and extremely comfortable to use. I needed to sleep on my back during recovery, and this pillow made it possible for me to get comfortable.

Non-Slip Socks or Slippers. My feet were cold, so I needed to keep them warm. We have slippery wood floors downstairs, and it was important that I didn't fall down when walking around. I could wear my non-slip socks all day and not worry about slipping if I went down the stairs.

Noise-Canceling Headphones. These were helpful in tuning out the homeschool noises going on downstairs. I wanted to jump in and solve problems, but that wouldn't help the family sort it out on their own. The headphones helped me enjoy the TV show I was watching and ignore all other distractions. I also used these during radiation when I was relaxing on the couch.

Simple Snacks. I needed to have some easy things to munch on in bed. I ate my meals downstairs, but sometimes I needed a snack. I enjoyed munching on healthy crackers that my kids would bring me in a little snack bowl.

Heating Pad. I had issues staying warm during the first few days after surgery. I got chills during my detox from the anesthesia and the pain medicine. I also got cold after my sponge baths. I would have the boys heat up a corn pad in the microwave, and I would place in on my legs or feet. I wasn't allowed to use it near my surgery site, but using it on my legs was helpful.

POST-SURGERY
STAYING AS COMFORTABLE AS POSSIBLE

There are many aspects to our well-being during the surgical recovery. The first part that I'm going to address is physical well-being. If we can take care of our bodies and feel comfortable, then we can expand our perspective to our mental and emotional well-being.

PAIN MANAGEMENT

One of the pieces of advice that I got from both my medical team and my dad was to stay ahead of the pain. If I let it get too unmanageable, I would need to take more medicine just to take the edge off.

I was nervous about post-surgery pain. A few years before, I had injured my shoulder while on vacation. I was unable to get relief for several weeks, and I was miserable. I made sure to discuss pain management with my surgeon before the lumpectomy.

He didn't think that I would be in too much pain because I wasn't having any lymph nodes removed, but he prescribed Tylenol with codeine just in case. As I mentioned before, I ended up working with Dave to manage my dosages.

I was only on the narcotic pain relievers for a few days. Even with such a short duration, I was already becoming physically dependent on the medication. To my surprise and distress, I got chills and shakes as I was tapering off the medication, even after such a short time.

As I said in chapter 7, there is a new method, called a nerve block, that is being used to help patients deal with the pain. Nerve blocks are injections that are given during surgery that block most of the immediate post-surgical pain. The nerve block will work for a few days after surgery and can help patients get through the most painful part of recovery.

Talk to your surgeon about pain management. If you are struggling, don't hesitate to reach out to your medical team. If they don't know how you are feeling, they can't offer you any help.

RISK OF INFECTION

Depending on your surgery, you may be prescribed antibiotics. It is important to keep an eye on the surgical area and be aware of any fever, redness, swelling, or increased pain. Your surgical team should have given you a list of the specific signs of infection to watch for. If you have any worrisome symptoms, place a call to your team.

SHOWERING

As I have spoken with many women, I have discovered that restrictions vary greatly with regard to showering. I had to wait over a week to have a proper shower because of my breast binding. I have talked to other women who were given clearance to take regular showers just a few days after their surgery.

The day after surgery, Dave helped me with my daily sponge baths. We would use the handheld showerhead to clean my lower body. Then I would wrap up in a towel and sit on a stool in the bathroom. Dave would unwrap me, one arm at a time, and clean me. That was humbling. I was cold, shivering, and felt like a child. I always felt so good after the sponge bath, but I didn't enjoy how I felt during them. Eventually, we decided to put a space heater in the bathroom to give extra warmth while I was getting my sponge bath.

Once I was cleared to shower, I was ecstatic—no more freezing sponge baths! But I needed to be extra careful about falling. One of the things I did was wear my Apple Watch on waterproof mode. Its fall detection mode would kick in if I slipped and fell and would notify my emergency contacts. If you don't have an Apple Watch or similar device, you might consider having someone nearby during your first few showers. Another way to keep safe in the shower is to use a shower chair.

If you have surgical drains, you can use a shower bag specially designed to hold them. Then you can clean yourself carefully, making sure not to disturb the area around the drains.

My hair needs to be washed every few days or it gets really greasy. So, a few days after my surgery, I had a professional wash and blow dry at the salon. It felt wonderful to get my hair clean and fluffed. I also had several bottles of dry shampoo that I would use in between shampoos.

RESTROOM

You might have difficulty wiping after your surgery, especially if you have had a mastectomy. Consider having wet wipes available for personal cleansing or install a handheld bidet. There are some bidets that can be easily installed on a standard toilet. A bidet can help you stay clean even when wiping is a challenge.

SLEEPING

As I mentioned before, my surgeon told me that I needed to sleep on my back until he cleared me for other positions. I am normally a side or stomach sleeper, so I had no idea how I would stay on my back. I purchased a wedge pillow that helped a lot. It was comfortable, and I was able to sleep soundly. Unfortunately for my husband, it didn't come with a snore suppressor.

Another option for sleeping would be a recliner. I've spoken with many ladies who loved their recliners for surgical recovery.

LIGHT PHYSICAL ACTIVITY

When I talked to my surgeon about what I could and couldn't do after surgery, he told me that anything that resulted in "breast bouncing" needed to be avoided. It is quite amazing how many activities will cause our breasts to move. I was told to limit walking to just what was necessary to get from one place in the house to another.

A few days after surgery, I started walking with Dave. I was feeling pretty good and wanted to get some fresh air. I told my surgeon about this activity during my first post-op appointment about a week after surgery. He said I needed to stop. Apparently, there were internal stitches in my breast and walking too much risked disturbing them. I wasn't happy, and I got quite stir crazy that second week of recovery.

You might have weight restrictions for lifting in place after your surgery. If you have children who are used to being picked up, you may need to prepare them for the changes during your recovery. Additionally, there may be restrictions on reaching for things above your head.

These restrictions frustrated me, especially as I was beginning to feel good. I was ready to start walking, but I didn't have clearance to do so. Instead, I did some stretching to regain my mobility.

STRETCHING

While I needed to keep my physical activity to a minimum, I also wanted to make sure I was doing stretches to help with mobility. One of the physical complications of breast cancer surgery can be a frozen shoulder. This is especially common with a mastectomy. A frozen shoulder is the loss of ability to move the shoulder due to inactivity. I had already dealt with shoulder pain, so I wanted to make sure that I didn't have this challenge in recovery.

I made sure to do some easy stretches right from the start. I would move my arms gently when I was walking around. I also did some recovery yoga. I searched online and found videos that were geared specifically for recovery from breast cancer surgery. When I first started doing these exercises, I would do them while lying down in my bed. There were videos that taught me how to do bed yoga. Later I moved to chair yoga.

I felt really good after stretching. This was one activity that I was able to do that wasn't going to bounce my breasts.

Another potential recovery challenge can be muscle cording. Muscle cords are long ropes of muscle that get tight during movement. This issue is common after procedures that biopsy or remove the lymph nodes. Stretching and physical therapy can reduce or eliminate this issue, but it can be painful. If you are having challenges with muscle cording, ask your surgical team for a referral to physical therapy.

CLOT PREVENTION

Blood clots can be a risk after surgery. I was instructed to get up and walk around a little bit every hour that I was awake. My Apple Watch was a great tool to help me remember. It would tap me if I hadn't gotten up in the previous hour. I would get up and walk slowly around my room for a minute or two. This was enough time to get my blood flowing and get my stand credit for the hour.

FALL RISK

I needed to be slow and careful when I changed positions after surgery. I got dizzy and needed time to adjust to standing up before I started walking. This challenge can be common after surgery. The discharge nurse made sure to give us a heads up about this risk so that we could take care at home to avoid falls.

For the first several days after surgery, the family would spot me on the stairs so that I didn't slip and fall.

CONSTIPATION

Anesthesia and pain medication will slow your bowels down. If you are having issues with constipation after surgery, you may consider taking something gentle to resolve the problem. Milk of Magnesia was recommended to me, but you may have different instructions. I ended up taking a wait-and-see approach and didn't need to take anything.

SURGICAL DRAINS

These are tubes with clear bulbs that may be placed inside the surgical area during your surgery. The purpose of the drains is to remove fluid from the area that is healing. These drains have specific care instructions. You may need to keep track of the color and amount of discharge. The drains will need to be emptied regularly and milked. You should receive instructions from your medical team.

There are special clothing items with pockets that can help you manage your surgical drains. It is also possible to pin the drains to your clothing to keep them in place.

Once the drainage slows down, your surgeon can remove the devices. This is usually done in the office during a post-op appointment.

It took some tweaking and adjusting to figure out the appropriate balance to stay physically comfortable during the first few weeks of my surgical recovery. I wasn't in excessive pain, for which I was grateful. However, I was mentally fatigued from the experience.

OTHERS' JOURNEYS
RECOVERY FROM SURGERY

Recovery is an individual process. In my interviews, I was struck with how different each woman's recovery from surgery was. It takes time to recover, physically and emotionally. Recovery is a process to work through and not a race that we must try to win. We can care for ourselves during this time by being patient with the healing that is taking place, both in our bodies and in our souls.

jill "The recovery was a little slow, I ended up with an infection on my right breast incision line as the surgeon had to take a lot from that area, so the closure was quite thin. I also developed blood clots in my lungs a month post-surgery which made my recovery that much slower. I will be on blood thinners for at least a year. Emotionally, I feel like I have weathered it okay. I have an incredibly supportive husband and a village of people around me, which helps tremendously. I would say get up and move whenever you can post-surgery, it helps physically and mentally, and make sure you have someone to talk to about how you are feeling; all feelings are valid. Give yourself time to grieve and heal."[1]

davita "I was very tired and sore the first week. I had incisions from hip to hip and of course the DMX incisions with the DIEP reconstruction. I was super emotional; losing your breasts will do that do you. Once the meds wore off, I was super agitated. I don't do well with sitting around. So I walked, a lot."[2]

jennifer f. "Recovery went smoothly after my initial hospitalization. My mom and daughters helped with showers and hair washing in the early days. It was so important to me to have their support. I did not want my husband to see my chest until after my drains were removed and bruising subsided. I also did not want him to be in a caregiver role given issues from my first marriage. Even after I had healed some though, it took him a while longer to be able to gather the strength to look. He has been nothing but loving and supportive but this process definitely took a toll on him, as well. I started walking within a few days of being home. At first, it was just to my driveway but each day I walked further. By time my drains came out on day 10, I was able to walk around the block twice. After the drains were removed, I increased my efforts, eventually making exercise a part of my daily routine. I believe it has helped me tremendously over the months and definitely recommend it."[3]

MENTAL WELL-BEING
BALANCING EFFORT & ENERGY

During the weeks of my surgical recovery, I needed to balance my mental effort with the energy level I had each day. I felt a significant amount of mental fatigue after surgery. I found it difficult to read books because I would lose focus quickly. I wasn't yet able to expend the mental effort. My mind would wander, and I would read the same sentence over and over again. Eventually, I would get frustrated and do something else.

Since I wasn't capable of reading, I ended up watching a lot of TV in my bed. Watching TV didn't take as much mental energy, and the shows helped me pass the time. During my treatment, I ended up watching all seven seasons of "The Mentalist." I finished the very last episode on my final day of radiation. I also used the shows to help me remember to get up. Once an episode finished, I would take a little walk around my room and then get comfortable for the next one.

I played a lot of puzzle and matching games on my iPad, as well. These types of games were relaxing and therapeutic. I also liked how these games helped me increase my mental stamina. Playing games was something that I could do to pass the time and challenge myself a little more each day.

As I continued to recover, I realized that there were some things that I could do to help out with the home management. I ended up working with Dave to plan meals and then place an online grocery order. He could stay home and monitor the virtual school while the shopping was done. I really enjoyed helping out with the shopping while I was recovering. It made me feel useful, even though I was sitting in bed! I could also pick out the snacks I wanted and make sure they got delivered.

I did need to learn how to balance my energy, especially when it came to visitors. I enjoyed having visitors, but I could only manage having one person come over a day. I had about an hour's worth of "visiting energy," and then I was too tired to make conversation. I had a chair set up in my room for my friends to sit in. This was helpful because we could chat and not disrupt the school going on downstairs.

Another thing that I enjoyed doing was talking on the phone. I liked having my phone calls before lunchtime. I had enough energy to enjoy the conversation, and then I could take a nap if I was tired.

I had expected and prepared myself for many of the physical challenges in recovery, but the mental and emotional ones were surprising. During one of our conversations, Dave helped me visualize my recovery in a very concrete way. He asked me to imagine a three-legged barstool. Each of the legs was one aspect of my well-being: physical, mental, and emotional. My recovery would be a process of rebuilding each of these legs. They wouldn't all recover at the same pace.

I really appreciated that visual. The imagery helped me put words to my recovery. When I was feeling strong emotions, I could talk about the emotional side of my recovery. If I was dealing with racing thoughts or focus issues, I was dealing with mental challenges. These were all valid components of my recovery.

EMOTIONAL WELL-BEING
ONE STEP FORWARD, TWO STEPS BACK

I was feeling pretty good a few days after my surgery. I asked Dave to come up and bring me a little snack. He did, and then I reached over and tried to give him a passionate kiss. I felt his lips tighten and his body pull away. After he went downstairs, I broke down sobbing. Was this our new normal?

I cried alone upstairs for a while. At first it was about the kiss. Then it was about my helplessness. I could hear life going on downstairs without me. I wasn't there to do my job. I didn't even know what my job was anymore.

Eventually, I decided to call Dave back up again. I don't think he was quite prepared for the mess that I was. I sobbed, and cried, and tried to put together some sentences. He sat on the bed next to me and let me get it all out.

He encouraged me to take the time I needed to heal. I had been through a big trauma over the last few months, and now that the surgery was done, all the emotions were welling to the surface. The lackluster kiss opened the floodgates. It was all coming out.

Things didn't get better overnight, but I did begin to acknowledge the emotional trauma I had been through. I had been through five biopsies, multiple imaging sessions, and a surgery. I needed to be present and put together to get through all of those procedures. Now, it was done, and I was feeling it all.

Gradually, I began to take steps to rebuild my emotional well-being. I enjoyed getting clean and brushing my hair every day. I would put on some pretty jewelry and comfortable clothes. My mom had sent me pretty pink slippers that I enjoyed wearing. I smiled every time I looked down at my sparkly feet. These small steps of self-care helped me feel better.

As I was sorting out my energy, emotions, and new physical challenges, I awaited the news as to whether the surgery successfully removed all of the cancer with clean margins. Was this lumpectomy my only one, or would I need a second surgery? I expected to hear the news at my surgical follow-up appointment.

The phone rang two days after my surgery. I looked down and saw an unknown number. I picked it up and heard my surgeon's voice, "Jennifer, I'm between surgeries, but I wanted to let you know that we got the pathology back, and the margins were clear!"

"Oh, my goodness, thank you so much for calling me!" I exclaimed. "Have a good day, and I'll see you at our appointment."

I hung up the phone, grateful and happy. There wasn't another surgery in my near future. Treatment wasn't finished, but the surgery was behind me.

10

THE BEAT GOES ON
oncology & post-surgical choices

THE PAPER GOWN CRINKLED. I swung my legs on the end of the exam bed and waited for my surgeon to enter the room. My mind raced, and my hair needed a good shampoo. It was eight days after my lumpectomy, and my breasts were still in the tight compression bandage. I hoped that today would be the day I got clearance to shower. I had no idea what I would look like after surgery, but I wasn't a huge fan of sponge baths.

I also hoped that I was healing quickly enough to move to the next phase of my cancer treatment. It was November 5, and I wanted to move treatment along as quickly as possible so that my insurance deductible didn't reset at the beginning of the year.

Cancer treatment is very expensive. Managing costs with insurance coverage is part of dealing with the business aspect of cancer. For the first time ever, we had hit our out-of-pocket maximum, and we weren't financially responsible for any of the new bills that came in. If I was going to do radiation, I wanted to maximize this benefit by getting my treatment finished before January.

MY JOURNEY
SURGICAL FOLLOW-UPS

I smiled at my surgeon when he walked in the room. The last time I had seen him had been right before surgery. He greeted me, took a look at my chart, and then walked over to unwrap the compression bandage. Once it was off, he looked closely at the incisions, then took a step back to evaluate the results. The surgeon said that I was healing well, then he turned to Dave and asked him what he thought.

That was awkward. Dave looked like a deer in headlights. He agreed with the surgeon, just to get the moment over with. Later, when I talked to Dave, he said that he had no idea how to respond. I was bruised, and the stitches were still in, as were markings from the pre-surgical planning. He had seen my breasts on better days.

My surgeon had the benefit of years of experience looking at breasts that were in various stages of recovery. His perspective was one of experience, while Dave and I were in shock at the trauma. It wasn't time to remove the stitches yet, but I did get clearance to shower. That was progress. He wanted to see me in a week to clip my stitches before he released me to oncology.

I put my bra back on, and we left for home. I was excited to get to shower again. Perhaps I would be able to wash some of the markings off. It would also give me a chance to see how I looked.

Once I got home, I went to take a look. It wasn't pretty. I was simultaneously thankful the surgery was over and apprehensive at how my breasts would look for the rest of my life. My breasts had been through trauma from the surgery and the biopsies. I was bruised and had black stitching on my incisions. I had no idea how I was going to heal, but at least I was going to be able to get clean.

I had two incisions, one on the right that removed the cancer. This one was on the outside of my breast and was about two inches long. The other incision was on my left breast and was about two inches above my nipple. The incision was about three-quarters of an inch long. This was where the surgeon had removed the benign fibroadenoma.

As I looked at myself, I began to second-guess my decisions. Did I really need to have that benign finding removed? I wasn't happy with how high up it was on my breast, and I was concerned about how it would heal. This scar bothered me for quite a while, especially since it took longer to fade than my cancer incision. At some point, I stopped thinking about the scars. I came to accept them and was thankful for the decisions that I made, but it took months for me to get to that point of acceptance.

A week later, two weeks after my lumpectomy, I had another appointment with my surgeon. He clipped the remaining stitches and said that I could begin with light exercise. Then he said, "Okay, I'll see you in six months. You can follow up with the oncologist to go over your pathology results and discuss any further treatment."

I was shocked. That was it. He was happy with the surgical results, and now we had moved to the follow-up phase. This felt strange because I had been seeing him regularly for months. I didn't expect to be released to oncology just a couple of weeks after my lumpectomy. But I was feeling better, and the incisions were healing well. My surgeon would order follow-up imaging for me for the next several years to monitor for a recurrence.

If you have had a mastectomy, there will likely be more extensive surgical follow-up in your future. The drains will need to be removed. Then, if you will have reconstruction, there will be regular fill appointments for your expanders. This procedure can be done by either your surgeon or your reconstructive specialist. It really depends on how your medical team likes to do things. Once the expanders are filled, then another surgery, called an exchange surgery, will be scheduled. If you have had DIEP flap reconstruction, there may be additional surgeries to address and adjust the cosmetic results.

The surgeon provided me a copy of my pathology during our last follow-up appointment. The next step was to make an appointment with an oncologist to determine treatment recommendations.

I walked out of my surgeon's office and went to the appointment counter to make an appointment with the oncologist. She asked, "I have an appointment in an hour with him. Would you like to take that one?"

"Absolutely!" I replied with a big grin on my face. I would be exhausted by the end of this day, but it would keep the treatment timeline moving. It was November 12, and there was no time to waste.

After she made the appointment, I returned to the waiting room. Dave handed me the pathology report and suggested that I start doing the research now to understand the results. No time like the present to get prepared for the appointment. This was going to be a long day!

TRANSITION TO ONCOLOGY

As I waited for my oncology appointment, I circled many sections of my pathology report. There were new words and complicated descriptions of the tissue removed in the document. I looked forward to getting my questions answered. A medical oncologist is a specialist in cancer treatment. Some oncologists specialize in certain cancer types. After breast cancer surgery, the oncologist will coordinate your treatment with other providers and plan your care using the pathology report from the surgery.

My oncologist worked in the same office as my breast cancer surgeon, and happened to be the first doctor that I had seen at the medical group. I was comfortable returning to him after my surgery. It was an easy choice to make.

SURGICAL PATHOLOGY REPORT

The oncologist will use the surgical pathology report to plan the next part of treatment. There are some cancers that can be treated with surgery alone. Breast cancer usually involves more treatment than just surgery. The treatments after surgery are designed to reduce the risk of a recurrence or of developing a second breast cancer.

The pathology report will include detailed information about what was removed during surgery. On the report, there will be details on margins, size, and weight of the sample.

It will also have information about biomarkers. These are what "feed" the cancer. The most common type of breast cancer is Hormone Receptor Positive (HR+). There are two types of receptors, estrogen and progesterone. The report will include information if the sample was ER+ or PR+. There will also be a percentage given next to these numbers indicating how much of the sample had these receptors. There will also be an indication if the tumor was HER2+, HER2-, or HER2 low. Breast cancers that test positive or low for this hormone tend to grow faster and can be more aggressive.[1]

Additionally, the cancer can be triple-negative or triple-positive. Triple-negative breast cancer is usually treated with chemotherapy because hormone treatments will not be effective. Triple-positive breast cancer has all three receptors and will require treatments that address all of these factors.

There are additional terms used to describe the combination of biomarkers in breast cancer. HR+/HER2- can also be called Luminal A. HR+/HER2+ can also be called Luminal B. The cancer biomarkers from your tumors will be used to design a custom treatment plan for you.

The pathology report will also include information about whether any lymph nodes tested positive for cancer. In my case, I didn't have any lymph nodes tested or removed during surgery. This is because my DCIS wasn't yet invasive.

Pathologists also describe the tumor based on how abnormal the cancer cells are. This is the grade of the cancer. Low-grade cancer indicates that most of the cells in the sample look like normal cells. Cancer can also be middle- or high-grade. In high-grade, the sample contains mostly cancerous cells. The grade of the cancer can be used to predict the potential spread of the cancer elsewhere in the breast.

All of this information will be combined to give the pathological prognositic stage of the cancer. This might be different from the clinical staging indicated by the biopsy because there are certain tests and information that can only be gathered after the surgery. The pathology report will include information in the TNM format.[2] T refers to the tumor size and location, N refers to the lymph node involvement, and M refers to the spread, or metastasis, of the cancer.

The pathological prognostic stage combines all information, including biomarker status, lab tests on tissue and lymph nodes, and additional clinical information. The stage will be given a number, and potentially a letter, to indicate the pathological stage of your cancer. This can range from 0 to IV.

Breast cancer staging is complicated. However, tumor size plays an important role in determining your pathological stage.[3] DCIS, and non-invasive Paget's disease of the breast (abnormal cells in the nipple) are considered stage 0 no matter what size they are. In stage I invasive cancer, the tumor size is less than 20 mm. Stage II invasive cancer tumors are between 20 and 50 mm. In stage III breast cancer, the tumor is larger than 50 mm. If the breast cancer has spread, or metastacized, outside the breast, it is considered Stage IV or metastatic. Each stage of breast cancer has different treatment protocols recommended either before or after surgery. As you look through your pathology report, I would take notes and then bring any specific questions up with your oncologist during your appointment.

DIAGNOSTIC TESTS TO PLAN POST-SURGICAL TREATMENT

In addition to the pathology report that will be sent to your oncologist, there may be additional tests ordered to determine your care plan. Some of these may be ordered as standard practice, but others may only be ordered at your request.

If there has been a diagnosis of invasive cancer and/or lymph node involvement, then there will likely be a test ordered that will help the oncologist determine the benefit of chemotherapy.

A sample of the tumor will be sent to a lab. Then a variety of genomic tests are run on the sample. The information received from these tests, along with your pathological information, will be used to give a score. This numerical score is a way of determining if chemotherapy would be appropriate. There are a couple of different types of this test. Some common ones include Oncotype and MammaPrint.

Talk to your oncologist to see if these tests will be run for you. In my case, since the cancer wasn't invasive, there was no reason to run them. However, there are a couple of tests that can be run on DCIS tumors to help plan for post-surgical treatment. These are not standard practice, and certain versions may not be covered by insurance.

I asked my oncologist to run the Oncotype DX Breast DCIS Score® test. This test would estimate the rate of recurrence that I would have if my DCIS was treated with surgery alone. It gave an estimated 10-year recurrence percentage of non-invasive and invasive cancer. There is another test called DCISionRT® that is designed to be a decision-making tool for radiation treatment. Its goal is to communicate the benefit of radiation to the patient. Certain patients will benefit more from radiation than others, and this test looks at information in the tumor that is linked to recurrence. This test wasn't available to me at the time of my diagnosis, so I wasn't able to ask about it. The only test that I knew about was the one available from Oncotype.

I received my Breast DCIS Score after I had already decided on doing radiation, but I'm glad that I asked for the test to be run. It added another piece of information to the puzzle of my DCIS and gave me confidence that I had made the right decision. My Breast DCIS Score was 27. That meant that my risk of local recurrence, of any kind, within 10 years was approximately 12 percent if treated with surgery alone. The risk of an invasive recurrence was 6 percent. This was on the low end of the risk scale. As I weighed my options, what stuck out to me was that these risk estimates were only 10-year options. I wanted to maximize my time without another breast cancer incident. That desire guided my post-surgical decisions.

Additional tests may be ordered to determine if there are circulating tumor markers remaining after treatment. These tests, which may be called liquid biopsies, may be ordered on a regular basis to see how well a treatment is working.[4]

If you are unsure what further treatments would be most beneficial to you, then I would talk to your oncologist and mention these tests. They could help with the decision-making process.

POST-SURGICAL TREATMENTS

After the oncologist has the appropriate information from pathology and the other diagnostic tests, it will be time to discuss recommendations for treatments after surgery. These can be radiation, hormone therapy, chemotherapy, or targeted treatments for HER2 positive cancer.[5]

FERTILITY

If you are considering having children in the future and would like to protect your fertility, it is important to discuss this with your oncologist before beginning any treatments. Cancer treatments may cause temporary or permanent infertility. Please take some time to have these hard conversations with your partner, if applicable, and with your medical team. In some cases, treatments can be modified to allow for future pregnancy. Some treatments, such as chemotherapy, can be done during pregnancy.

RADIATION

Radiation therapy is typically recommended to patients who have undergone a lumpectomy since there may be cancer cells left in the breast that have not yet been detected with imaging.

The most standard type of radiation therapy targets the whole breast with an external radiation beam. Another option for radiation is partial-breast radiation. This treatment targets only the area of the breast impacted by cancer. There is also internal radiation therapy, brachytherapy, which is targeted just to the tumor area. The device that delivers this type of therapy is placed inside the breast and delivers radiation from the inside out.[6]

ENDOCRINE (HORMONE) THERAPY

Most breast cancers are hormone receptor-positive, meaning that the estrogen and progesterone that our bodies produce naturally are feeding the growth of the cancer cells. There are a variety of oral medications that can be prescribed to reduce the amount of estrogen in the body and lower the risk of breast cancer returning.[7] The type of medication depends on your menopausal state at diagnosis. These medications are usually prescribed for 5-10 years. The benefit of the medication will persist even when it is stopped.

If you are pre-menopausal, you will be prescribed a medication that will reduce the amount of estrogen that your breast tissue absorbs. This type of drug is called a selective estrogen receptor modulator (SERM). Tamoxifen, the most commonly prescribed SERM, has been approved for over 40 years to reduce the risk of a breast cancer recurrence. It can also be taken before a breast cancer diagnosis in patients who are considered high risk.

If you are post-menopausal, there is another class of medications that will be prescribed. These are called aromatase inhibitors. These will block the residual estrogen that is produced in fat tissues. There are several different types available. If you have a hard time with the side effects on one, it is possible to switch medications. Many women said that switching medication helped them better tolerate the medicine.

Another option to reduce the amount of estrogen in the body is to suppress the ovaries. The ovaries are the primary source of estrogen in pre-menopausal women. They can either be removed surgically (if the woman is not planning on having children) or suppressed via medication.

All the treatment options will reduce the amount of estrogen in the body. There are side effects that mimic some of the menopausal symptoms women have. These may include:

- Hot flashes
- Bone pain
- Depression and mood challenges
- Headache
- Hair thinning
- Vaginal dryness
- Loss of sexual desire
- Weight changes
- Nausea
- Sleep issues
- Endometrial cancer
- Pulmonary embolism
- Blood clots
- Cognitive decline

I was concerned about some of the side effects that I might have while on tamoxifen. I was especially concerned about the risk of weight gain, depression, and sexual side effects. During my first appointment with my oncologist, I had a lengthy discussion with him about my concerns. He listened, and then had some advice that really helped. He suggested that I try taking the tamoxifen. I should reach out to him as I experienced side effects, and we would work on strategies to address them. He also said that if the side effects were really bad, I could just stop taking it. I was in charge of this part of my treatment. If it impacted my quality of life, and I wasn't functioning well, I should stop taking it.

That encouragement was what I hung on to as I began taking the tamoxifen. I started taking it in January 2020 once I was done with radiation. I had some side effects that came on immediately. I got hot flashes, and I was moody. Then, the vaginal dryness came on. After a month or so, the hot flashes and mood issues resolved. I was able to manage the vaginal dryness with lubricant, which I'll talk about in the upcoming chapter on sex.

I was on tamoxifen for about nine months and then I began to get rib pain. My oncologist thought that it might be because of working out. But when it didn't go away for a while, I did some additional research. As I read through the list of common and uncommon side effects, I found a listing for rib pain as a rare side effect.[8] That was enough to encourage me to message my oncologist again. He recommended I stop taking tamoxifen for a while and see what happened. The rib pain went away once I stopped. When I went back on after a few weeks, the pain gradually came back. I messaged my oncologist again, and he recommended that I stop taking it so that I wasn't dealing with the pain on an everyday basis. In my case, the tamoxifen would provide a reduction of risk of getting breast cancer in the opposite breast but didn't have a life-saving benefit for me as a DCIS patient.[9]

I had mixed emotions about stopping the tamoxifen. I felt like a failure because I couldn't tolerate the side effects. Should I have toughed it out over the next four years with a constant stitch in my side? I thought back to my initial conversation with my oncologist when he told me that we could work together to make sure that I maintained a good quality of life while on the medication. Taking me off the tamoxifen allowed me to get through the day without rib pain. I remember talking with Dave as I was going off the tamoxifen, and he said to me, "Do you have any reason not to trust your oncologist about this?" I racked my brain and realized that I didn't. I trusted him and his judgement in this situation.

I'm glad that I tried the tamoxifen. I was able to be on it for about 11 months. If I hadn't had the rib pain, I would have kept taking it, despite the other systemic side effects. Those were manageable. I am grateful that my oncologist was willing to work with me about the challenges of endocrine therapy. He never dismissed my concerns or minimized my side effects. I appreciated that.

CHEMOTHERAPY & TARGETED THERAPIES

Chemotherapy can be added on as a post-surgical treatment if the cancer is invasive and has spread to the lymph nodes. Triple-negative cancer is also usually treated with chemotherapy. There are a variety of chemotherapy drugs which are highly effective at treating breast cancer.

As I mentioned before in the pathology section, a test such as Oncotype may be ordered after your surgery to determine if chemotherapy will be recommended for your particular tumor. The results from this test can take several weeks to receive since the samples need to be sent to specific labs for analysis.

There are also special targeted treatments available that are designed for HER2-positive breast cancer. These are usually done as an infusion or via an injection every three weeks for a year. Adding this targeted treatment to chemotherapy can dramatically reduce the risk of recurrence.

If you are facing chemotherapy or infusions for HER2 breast cancer after surgery, I highly recommend picking up some other books that can offer you more information about the types of drugs used, supplemental therapies to minimize side effects, and support and encouragement for this treatment. I'll include a few recommended resources in the appendix.

OTHERS' JOURNEYS
CHEMOTHERAPY

Some of the women I interviewed had chemo as a part of their treatment. Here are a few of their experiences and tips for getting through this phase of the journey.

noelle Chemo before surgery. "I had neoadjuvant (preoperative) chemotherapy. I was diagnosed March 30 and started chemo April 17. It all happened very fast, but I was eager to start fighting this beast. Because my cancer was HER2-positive and very aggressive, they wanted to attack it aggressively with chemo before any surgery was performed."[10]

davita Chemo after surgery. "[Chemo] was not part of the original plan. After surgery, my pathology report showed it was aggressive and high in estrogen as well as larger than they thought. I had four months of aggressive chemo. Helpful tip: Listen to your body. Everyone is different. Do what you feel you can so you don't just sit around all the time. Movement is needed and drink lots of fluids. Everyone pushes water but some people can't tolerate it; just drink fluids."[11]

jill Had multiple types of chemo before and after surgery. "Chemotherapy is different for everyone, but one thing that helps everyone is hydrating! Hydrating makes all the difference. Make sure to drink as much water as you can to help flush the chemo from your system. Educate yourself, join support groups for your specific cancers and the drugs you will be taking. It helps because the side effects are relatively universal to degrees, and you have an amazing group of people rooting you on through it!!"[12]

jennifer f. Had chemo after surgery. "After surgery, I learned my tumor had spread to at least one lymph node as well as my chest wall. . . I was not expecting to need chemotherapy given we thought the tumor was still stage I so it was another upsetting setback . . .Try to maintain a positive outlook whenever possible. I struggled with chemotherapy thinking I was injecting myself with poison. That negativity affected how I felt. I found a meditation (on YouTube) for chemo patients reframing chemotherapy drugs as medicine. I stopped thinking I was going in to be poisoned and instead looked at it as I was going in to be healed. We cannot change the position we find ourselves in so it is important to try and find the positives where you can."[13]

janelle Decided to use cold cap to preserve her hair during chemo. "The decision to cold cap was a very difficult one, due to the expense, how labor intensive it is on chemo infusion days and lots of hair care rules. Even though my chemo occurred during the COVID shutdown, and I could have easily hid my bald head from the world, I ultimately decided to do it for my kids. I wanted life to be as normal as possible for them. Cold capping brought me a sense of normalcy when it felt like the world around me was crashing down."[14]

MENTAL WELL-BEING
PROCESSING INFORMATION

As much as the diagnostic process stretched my research skills, I actually found the post-surgery choices more overwhelming. I knew that surgery to remove the breast cancer was required, but what choices should I make about my post-surgical care? The more I researched, the more I felt myself becoming overwhelmed. I wanted to be an informed patient, but I also didn't want to worry and feel anxious about what the perfect choice would be.

To participate in this process as best as possible, we need to avoid information overload. I would recommend asking for printed copies of your pathology reports. These might be available in your patient portal already but, in my case, I needed to ask for the hard copies. I liked having the paper reports because I could look through them and mark up my questions.

On the day that I transitioned from surgery to oncology, I used the time between appointments to look over my pathology report and make notes of my questions right on the paper. This helped me know what questions I had and guided the conversation.

If you have time to prepare before your oncology appointment, I recommend writing down the questions you have beforehand so that you can take advantage of the time during the appointments.

Another thing that was challenging for me during this transition was decision fatigue. I had the choice to take the tamoxifen. I could decide to skip radiation if I wanted to. I had to be careful to avoid letting my decision-making drift into mental anxiety.

One of the things that helped me was that the oncologist was willing to work with me on these post-surgical choices. He would monitor me and be available to answer any questions that came up during treatment. I was glad that he was willing to work with me to address my rib pain and to recommend that I stop treatment because of the issue.

If chemotherapy is recommended, there will be blood work ordered to make sure that each treatment is safe for you. Additionally, you will be monitored during the infusions by a medical team to watch for any adverse reactions. Oncologists can stop or modify a treatment protocol if it is causing too many other medical issues.

I tried to take care of my mental well-being by limiting my processing time for the medical information. I did a little research every day, and then stopped when I got tired. I was able to educate myself on the treatments without exhausting myself. I also made sure to reach out to my care team when issues came up.

EMOTIONAL WELL-BEING
A LONG PATHWAY TO ACCEPTANCE

Many emotions can come up after the initial period of surgical recovery. It can be a shock when we first see ourselves after surgery. It certainly was for me. I didn't know if I would ever get to the point where I would be okay with the new scars.

It takes time to process the change to or loss of our breasts. One of the things that I did to address the emotions I felt when I was getting dressed was to be conscious of the thoughts I was thinking. If I felt frustrated about my new scars, I would actively replace that thought with gratitude that the cancer was removed. It took months before those mental affirmations became a habit.

I also had plenty of anxiety and fear heading into radiation and endocrine therapy. I was nervous about the treatments and side effects. I was just starting to feel physically better after all the biopsies and the surgery, and I still wasn't done. I was emotionally and physically exhausted. I just wanted to be done with treatment. However, I had a month of radiation ahead of me and a goal to get it done before the new year. There was no time to take a break from cancer treatment.

11 RADIATION
bring headphones

BEFORE I LEFT MY oncology appointment, I asked the doctor for a referral to a radiation center. Radiation treatment is commonly recommended after a lumpectomy to eliminate any additional cancer cells left in the breast. I was pretty sure that I would do radiation and wanted to get the treatment started as soon as possible so that I could be done before Christmas and the insurance deductible reset on January 1.

Radiation was a significant part of my DCIS treatment. In this chapter, I'll share why I decided to do radiation, what it was like for me to go through it, and what kinds of side effects I experienced. It wasn't an easy treatment to walk through, but I'm glad I opted to do it.

MY JOURNEY
MEETING MY RADIATION ONCOLOGIST

I had no idea what to expect when I walked in for my radiation consult. It was a new office and a different medical group. We had chosen a nearby center to make the potential transportation to and from daily treatment as short as possible. As I sat in the waiting room, I thought about what might happen during the consult. I was pretty sure I would be headed into an exam room.

Instead, Dave and I were called into a consultation room with some chairs and no exam table in sight. I was a little confused. After some conversations with the nurse, the radiation oncologist walked in. She was carrying her tea and greeted us with a warm smile. Her demeanor was calm, friendly, and confident.

She began the consult with a brief summary of my treatments thus far. Without any notes in front of her, she was able to tell my entire story back to me: all the biopsies, the imaging, the surgery, and the pathology of my cancer. She stopped a few times to make sure that she had the order right. When she was done, she said, "Well, you have certainly had quite the diagnosis and treatment so far."

I'm not quite sure if my jaw dropped visibly, but it certainly did in my head. She had clearly read all my medical records and was well prepared for this appointment. If this was going to be the doctor responsible for my radiation treatment, she had quickly earned my trust. I felt she would be an excellent person to plan and follow this next part of my treatment.

NEW CARE PROVIDER
THE RADIATION ONCOLOGIST

Radiation oncologists are specialists in designing and delivering radiation to cancer patients. They work alongside a team to plan treatments that are as effective as possible while minimizing damage to surrounding tissue. The location, angle, and dosage of radiation all need to be precisely calculated for the treatment to be most effective. These doctors take additional training for at least five years to become board certified.[1]

The radiation oncologist will plan and calculate the treatment and participate with the mapping for most effective delivery. Once this preliminary stage is complete, the additional members of the radiology team will be responsible for the daily treatments. You will see the oncologist regularly to discuss side effects and manage the treated area.

CHOOSE A CONVENIENT TREATMENT LOCATION IF POSSIBLE

Radiation is usually a daily treatment for several weeks. My treatment was 20 sessions that were divided into segments of five treatment days and two rest days over the weekend. Treatments can vary in length depending on the individual diagnosis.

When you are considering radiation treatment, I highly recommend choosing a location that is close and convenient to your home or work. You may need to ask for a referral to a different medical group, as I did, to make treatment more convenient for you and your caregivers. If you live in a remote area and travel will present a hardship, it may be possible to work with a charitable organization or a nearby hospital to arrange for housing during the week.

The actual radiation treatment sessions are about 15 minutes long, so if you can minimize the travel time, it will allow you to have more time in your day for resting.

RADIATION PREPARATION APPOINTMENTS

Because radiation treatment is customized for each person, planning and simulation appointments are needed so that the equipment can be calibrated for your diagnosis. I had three separate appointments before my treatment began. Your office might do things slightly differently.

INITIAL CONSULTATION

My first appointment was the initial consultation with my radiation oncologist. This appointment was a chance for me to have an extended conversation about whether this treatment would be beneficial for me.

One of the topics that I brought up was whether radiation would be an appropriate treatment, especially since my DCIS was only four millimeters in size and was removed with clear margins. Would it be appropriate for me to undergo radiation for such a small amount of cancer?

My oncologist gave two reasons for recommending I pursue treatment. The first reason was my age. I was 41 at diagnosis, and she hoped that I would have another 40 years of life ahead of me. Having plenty of life ahead of me meant more time for cancer cells to grow. There are some new recommendations that indicate that patients over 70 at diagnosis can safely skip radiation after a successful removal of the cancer.[2]

The second reason she brought up was that radiation would eliminate any cancer cells in my breast that hadn't yet been detected in imaging. My cancer was slow growing and had likely been there for years before it was detected. It was possible I had other cancerous areas in my breast that weren't large enough to show up on imaging. According to my radiation oncologist, radiation would "reset" the breast and take care of any of those rogue cells.

Another thing to discuss at this initial appointment would be the potential side effects that are most concerning to you. As you research side effects, it can feel overwhelming to think about all of them. One thing to consider as you read through the lists of side effects is that not everyone experiences all of them at once. In my case, I had fatigue and skin peeling. These were not pleasant, but they were manageable. It helped immensely that the oncologist was willing to listen and talk about my fears and concerns.

There are different ways of delivering the radiation during treatment.[3] I had CT-guided radiation, or tomotherapy. This is a newer technique that takes a CT image of you before each radiation session and uses this to map up to a stored image of your body. It allows for precise aiming of the radiation beams to avoid any other organs. The radiation was delivered to me while I was in a circular tunnel—a little like an MRI tube. Other radiation treatments may be done in an open room with the machine moving around you.

Depending on the location of your tumor, there may be some other unique concerns that need to be addressed before treatment. Since our breasts are so close to our heart and lungs, it is important to protect them during treatment. Radiation oncologists can do this by careful positioning of the radiation beams and other techniques like breath holds during treatment. Talk to your practitioner about what she plans to do to protect your other organs from damage.

Another component of this consultation may be a physical examination by your radiation oncologist. She will look at your breasts and make sure that you are healed enough from surgery to undergo treatment. In my case, I was able to start radiation about four weeks after my lumpectomy. This examination will also help her make her initial planning for your treatment. Once you decide to undergo treatment, another appointment will need to be scheduled to plan out the specifics of your radiation.

RADIATION PLANNING & MAPPING APPOINTMENT

My radiation planning and mapping appointment was scheduled several days after my initial consultation. This appointment was two hours long and involved many different steps. It was the longest appointment that I had during my radiation treatment.

I began the appointment by going into the treatment room. The techs had me lie down on the table. The radiation oncologist came in and the team began to make plans on how it would be best to have me positioned for the appointment. The radiation oncologist used a marker to draw on me. She made an outline of my breast tissue and they used the outline to plan out areas for the radiation tattoos.

I was not excited that I would need to get tattoos for this treatment. I was concerned that they would be visible long after my radiation was finished. I decided to take time to ask questions before they placed them. I'm happy I did because it allowed me to eliminate a marking that I thought would be visible after treatment. After discussing my concerns with the team, they decided to use my existing freckles and moles as a part of their locating technique. I ended up with only one radiation tattoo on my side.

The radiation tattoos are the size of a small freckle and are dark purple. The tool they used to mark me was kind of like a pen with a sharp tip. It was pretty fast and not too painful.

During my planning appointment, the team created a mold for a custom pillow that I would lie on. The pillow would position me precisely at a slight angle for every treatment. At the end, I worked with my techs to "deflate" my pillow and celebrate.

I also had CT imaging done during this mapping appointment. This CT image would be the template that would help plan my treatment and ensure that I was in the correct position each time for my radiation treatment. At every session, another image was taken of me and matched up to the CT on file. This ensured precise delivery of the radiation.

Another part of this planning will be to record your weight because radiation doses need to be precisely calibrated to measure the toxicity of treatment. You will be measured weekly to ensure that the dosage remains appropriate.

Once the planning session is done, the team will work together to produce a treatment schedule for you. I would have twenty sessions of radiation and one simulation appointment. As I mentioned before, a typical radiation schedule will be five days on and two days off. In my case, because my treatment began near Thanksgiving, I would come in for my first treatment on the Sunday before Thanksgiving and only have four treatments during that week. This type of modification is typical around holidays.

RADIATION SIMULATION APPOINTMENT

I came in for my simulation appointment about a week after my mapping appointment. This was a dress rehearsal for the team and an opportunity for me to get an idea of what the treatments would be like. The techs showed me where to pick up my gown and where to put my things. They showed me the secondary waiting room that I would sit in until my treatment time. Once they were ready for me, they walked me through the actual appointment procedures.

I got positioned on the radiation table just as I would be during my treatment appointments. The team ran through the imaging part of the procedure to make sure their CT scans taken during the planning session matched up to what they were seeing that day. After my simulation was complete, I was ready to begin the actual treatments in just a few days.

TREATMENT TIME

I arrived at the office on my first treatment day full of nerves. After checking in with the receptionist, I walked through the doors and into the changing area. I picked out a gown and went into the dressing rooms. I put it on, locked my clothes and purse in the locker, and went to sit in the secondary waiting room. There was soft music playing in the background and pretty fall decorations on the wall.

Right on time, the techs called me back to the treatment room. They greeted me warmly and had me get onto the table. My custom mold was already there along with a sheet, which helped the techs position me. The room was freezing! "Would you like a warm blanket?" one of the techs asked.

"Yes, please!" I responded. I laid down on the table and they had me unwrap my gown to ensure correct positioning. There were red lights in the ceiling which served as guiding beacons. I was told to hold still. The techs moved me slightly using the sheet underneath me. Once they were confident in the positioning, they covered me up again and put a warm blanket over my legs. It was time for the treatment to start.

The techs left the room but told me that they were always available and listening if I had any issues or got uncomfortable. They would stop treatment if I called out to them. After the door closed, I felt the radiation table move into the tube, and the scan began. The first part of my treatment each time was a positioning CT scan. The scan didn't take long, and the table moved out again. I thought, "Hey, that wasn't bad. Am I done?" Then I heard the machine start to warm up again. There were rattling and tapping sounds coming from the tube.

The table moved me back into the rattling tube. The tapping sounds continued and began making circles around me. Panic swept over me, and I willed myself to hold still. How long was this going to last? I didn't want to move and mess things up, but I was freaking out inside.

After what seemed like ages, the rattles slowed down and the table moved out again. I held still, not knowing what was next. I breathed a huge sigh of relief when the door opened, and the techs came in. I sat up and told them that I was really frightened by the noises. They told me the noises were normal and that I was welcome to bring headphones to wear during treatment.

I left the treatment room, 5 percent done with my radiation, grateful I had made it through that first session. I didn't want to panic throughout all the treatments, so I decided that I needed music to distract me. It was Christmas season, and the machine sounded like rats, so I decided on the *Nutcracker* soundtrack. I had danced in that ballet as a child, and I love the music. This would be a festive way for me to get through treatment each day.

If your radiation treatment isn't CT-guided, the radiation delivery system may be done with a stationary table and a device circling around you. The delivery isn't painful. In fact, I didn't feel anything physically during treatment. It was the mental part that was difficult in the office.

I found that it was easier for me to get through treatment by closing my eyes, concentrating on my breathing, and listening to music. I tried to visualize myself dancing in the ballet or lying on a beach enjoying the tropical breezes. I didn't like opening my eyes because the top of the tube was above me, and I can have issues with claustrophobia. I was able to avoid that by closing my eyes.

I would bring a small bag with me that included lotion, deodorant, and thermal water. Before I changed into my clothes, I would take time to care for my skin. I would spray on the thermal water, gently pat my breast dry with the treatment robe, then put on some lotion. I would also put on my deodorant. There may be restrictions on when you can put lotion and deodorant on, so follow the instructions given to you by the office.

I was usually in the office for about a half an hour total. I would get there about ten minutes early to get changed. Treatment would take around fifteen minutes and then I was free to head home. My appointments were longer once a week because I would see the radiation oncologist.

These weekly radiation oncology appointments would be right after my treatment for the day. First, I would get weighed and then head into an exam room. The nurse would ask me about my side effects and address any concerns I had. Then the radiation oncologist would come in. I would talk to her about any side effects I was experiencing. Then she would take a look at my skin and make sure that it was coping okay with the treatment. If the skin effects begin to get bad, the radiation oncologist can prescribe creams that will help or put a pause on your treatment to allow your skin to recover.

I was anxious and scared for my first treatment, but gradually I was able to get into a routine. I got to know the radiation techs and enjoyed the small talk before and after. Then I would head home to cope with the side effects.

COMMON SIDE EFFECTS WITH RADIATION

I experienced two primary side effects during my radiation treatment: fatigue and skin peeling. Your side effects may be different. I have talked with women who never burned at all and who weren't tired. That was not the case for me.

FATIGUE

During my month of radiation treatment, our family would finish eating dinner, and my eyes would glaze over in exhaustion. It was 6:30, and I was no longer able to have conversations with my family. Dave would look over at me and encourage me to go up to bed. It was common for me to be in my pajamas relaxing in bed by 7 p.m. during my radiation treatment. It was as if all the energy had been sucked out of me. I would fall asleep early, usually by 8:30 or 9, and sleep deeply.

Fatigue was the most challenging side effect for me. A good night of sleep would help me have more energy in the mornings, but it was not close to my pre-radiation levels. I got increasingly tired the longer I was in treatment. That is normal and to be expected. The fatigue tends to be cumulative in radiation treatment.[4]

I tried to work with the physical energy I had rather than spending time getting frustrated that I was exhausted. The physical fatigue was a sign that my body was trying to heal itself. The best way I could support myself was to rest and recuperate. I used a timer to limit the length of my physical activities. Doing this allowed me to get some things done, and then rest after. I also tried to take at least one slow walk a day. Walking and light physical activity have been shown to reduce fatigue in radiation patients. It seems counterintuitive, but it worked for me. I walked in the morning because that was when I had the most energy.

My energy began to return when treatment finished. One night, about a week after, I was lying in bed, totally awake, and listening to the movie that the guys were watching downstairs. I came down in my pajamas and joined them. The evening fog had lifted, and I was able to return to my standard bedtime routine.

SKIN BURNING & PEELING

I hate sunburns. When I'm on vacation, I am diligent about using sunscreen. If I can avoid a burn, I will. By the time I was about halfway through treatment, my right breast looked like I had fallen asleep on a topless beach and forgotten to put any sunscreen on. It was the worst burn that I ever had.

I was able to use creams and take special care of my skin to minimize the discomfort. In many ways, it looked worse than it felt.

I began applying creams right away. I started with the recommended creams from my radiation team. They had samples available and had also given me a list of other ones I could try. Most of them were available at Target or Amazon, but I purchased the Calendula at my local Sprouts. There are also prescription creams that might be recommended for you. As your skin begins to get more sensitive, it might become necessary to try a different cream in the middle of treatment. I used Calendula at the beginning but needed to move to Aquaphor once my skin started to peel.

It is essential that you clear all your creams with your oncologist. Some creams, such as ones which contain antioxidants, cannot be used during treatment because they will make the radiation less effective.

In addition to creams, I also needed to take special care of my skin by choosing clothing that didn't irritate the treatment area. I wore soft clothing and bras that were made of soft material. Some patients have shared that going braless helped them. I tried that, but it made the itching much worse.

I was also told to avoid temperature extremes on my breasts. That meant no extremely hot showers, hot tubs, or ice packs. When I was in the shower, I used very gentle soap and tried not to let the water directly hit my breasts. I gently patted my skin dry, avoiding any rubbing on the area. It is really important not to pick the areas that are peeling. Keep them clean and dry and watch for signs of infection.

My right breast peeled completely two times: once in the middle of treatment and again several weeks after treatment finished. The skin darkened and turned purple. Then it peeled off. It was uncomfortable when my nipple began to peel. I used Aquaphor on it to minimize the sensitivity and discomfort. I continued to apply lotion regularly for several weeks after the peeling stopped. My skin was darker than normal for quite a while after treatment finished, but it eventually returned to its normal shade.

There are other side effects that are possible during radiation treatment. If you have any concerns about whether what you are experiencing is normal or not, reach out to your treatment team for guidance. They are great resources for information and should be able to help you manage the side effects of radiation.

OTHERS' JOURNEYS
RADIATION EXPERIENCES & TIPS

If there was one thing I heard consistently in my interviews about radiation treatment, it was to "stay moisturized." Following this advice can help us stay comfortable. I remember feeling exhausted with cancer treatment before I started radiation, and then even more so once it started. Sometimes, as we are transitioning to a new treatment, emotions bubble up, as they did for Joni.

joni "I did my staging for radiation and lost it. I asked that they get my husband because I couldn't stop crying. I guess I'd been blocking everything, and it hit me all at once.

My go-to was a lot of Aquaphor. I wore two tops, one was a thin spaghetti strap in black or dark blue to put over my greased-up skin and I would fold up the top under my breast to keep my breast dry. I would then put any top I wanted over that so I didn't get lotion or grease on it. It worked out great. I had no stains on my lighter-colored top and I kept dry."[5]

nancy "My advice is to stay hydrated and be generous applying lotion during radiation treatment and after. Stay [out] the sun as much as possible. Also, stretching to prevent or help with skin tightness is important once the skin has healed."[6]

nanci "If you think you've put enough cream on, you haven't, apply more. Also, larger breasted women can tend to get a heat rash under the radiated breast. Cut a soft cotton T-shirt in strips and place a strip under the breast to help prevent rubbing and the irritation and pain associated with this."[7]

MENTAL WELL-BEING
DEALING WITH THE MENTAL FATIGUE & LOGISTICS

In addition to being physically exhausted during radiation, I was also mentally exhausted. I found it difficult to focus on anything for a long time. I would try to read a book and wasn't able to get more than a few pages into it before I was too tired.

I accommodated my short attention span by doing my "thinking work" in short bursts. I would set aside fifteen minutes to do any research or reading that I needed, and then I would take a break. I also tried to write things down so that I didn't forget them. The mental fog began to lift once I finished active treatment and was feeling less physically fatigued.

Radiation was five days a week and that meant that I needed to schedule my life around it. The most important hour of every day was my radiation time. It was the holidays and that meant extra opportunities to see family and fellowship at church, but I was too exhausted to participate. I had to decline social invitations during radiation because my priorities were treatment and virtual school supervision. I didn't have energy for anything else. We would leave for my radiation appointment each day at 2:20 for my 2:45 appointment. On most days, I was back home from treatment by 3:30.

Dave went back to work during radiation but was able to take me to my treatments almost every day. On the days that he couldn't take me, I asked a neighbor to drive me. Since I was experiencing so much fatigue, it was better for me to get a ride to and from treatment.

Another component of my mental well-being was managing my thoughts. As I was lying on the table during the sessions, I thought about how paradoxical this was. I was allowing the doctors to radiate me just enough to kill the cancer, but not enough to kill me. Those thoughts didn't help very much with my anxiety, so I tried to limit them and think about other things.

Acknowledging the power of the treatment helped me accept my fatigue more. I might have looked fine from the outside, but my insides were battling this treatment. If I needed to go to bed early to rest, then it was okay.

EMOTIONAL WELL-BEING
ACCEPTING A SEASON OF EMOTIONAL EXHAUSTION

It took all of my energy to get through the treatments each day. When I got home, I was exhausted and sapped. This was much more than physical and mental exhaustion. I had no emotional energy at all. I would zone out and disengage at the dinner table. My boys would be chattering on with Dave about their day, and I was unable to participate. I was physically present, but emotionally unavailable.

I also really struggled with guilt during this time. One of the most difficult and emotional decisions was to stay home for Thanksgiving. We had received an invitation from Dave's sister to come over for the holiday, but it was right after I started treatment. I was concerned about how tired I would be after a holiday celebration. I remember crying tears of frustration that my treatment was impacting our family so much. It was the right decision, but it was such an emotional one to make.

Another emotion that I struggled with was anger about how hard this was for me. Occasionally, I would hear stories from others that radiation was "no big deal" for them. They were able to go on with their daily life, take an hour for treatment, and then jump right back in. I was saying no to things left and right and struggling to get through the day. I would get angry because it was so hard.

We will all have unique experiences with side effects from treatments. There doesn't appear to be any rhyme or reason to the variability. I've spoken to fair-skinned women who never had their skin peel or turn red. Some women can continue working throughout, and others, like me, experience severe fatigue.

There is no "right" way to be a cancer patient. The surgeries, treatments, and recovery will look and feel different for all of us. If you are sailing through radiation, that is great. And if you are dragging yourself to each appointment, that is okay, too.

I grew excited as I approached the end of my radiation treatment. This would mark the completion of active treatment, and I was looking forward to a new year with new adventures. Each day I would come home and mark an "x" on my calendar.

December 23, 2019 was my last day of radiation. It had been three months since my cancer diagnosis. I walked into the office, feeling excited to be done. I wasn't sure what the traditions were at my office for completing treatment. Other survivors told me about ringing a celebratory bell at the end, but this office had none. There is much debate as to whether the tradition of bell ringing is sensitive and appropriate for an end-of-treatment celebration. There are patients for whom treatment will not end, and they won't ever ring the bell.

Since I wasn't exactly sure what the office did to celebrate, I improvised my own celebratory ritual. I decided to ask my tech if he would let me deflate my radiation pillow. He looked at me and said that he had never had a patient ask to do that before. After my last session, he came in and we used the machine to deflate it. The other techs handed me a little bell and played a song for me. I ran around the office with more energy than I had showed in months. Everyone in the office laughed and celebrated with me. I had Dave take pictures of me with my team, and then I got changed for the last time.

It was surreal to walk out of the radiation treatment center and know that I was done. My active treatment had finished. I was burned and exhausted. Christmas was in two days. I didn't care what was under the tree. Finishing treatment was the best present that I could have asked for!

12

BREAST CANCER SWIRL

handling complex post-treatment emotions (yours & theirs)

FINISHING RADIATION WAS A huge milestone. For months, our family schedule had revolved around my appointments. Suddenly, it was all done. I was filled with hope but also hesitation. My dad had told me this, as I approached the end of treatment, "Sometimes it can be harder to deal with the cancer once treatment is finished. When you're in treatment, you're doing something active to fight it. But, when it's done, there's nothing else to do." The echo of those words rang in my memory as I walked out of treatment and into the next phase of my life.

Cancer treatment, no matter what your stage, is hard. We need to push ourselves to get through. Then it finishes, and we are left with the memories. We can feel the full weight of what we have been through. It is completely normal to feel a wide range of emotions when active treatment finishes. We don't need to be happy all the time.

There is a medically recognized form of post-treatment trauma in cancer patients.[1] Certain smells, sounds, or memories can bring us right back to the scary moments of treatment. When I first walked back into the mammogram room for my six-month imaging, I felt a wave of anxiety. It was like I was reliving the cancer diagnosis again.

Survivorship is a complicated process. While our active treatment has finished, our recovery hasn't.

I was excited to finish up treatment, but I was nervous about what it would look like for me to begin taking over my job again. I was extremely fatigued from radiation and wasn't sure how I was going to make it through the day. Just a few weeks after I completed radiation, Dave returned to business travel, and the kids returned to school after winter break. Life was returning to normal, but my mind and body were still recovering.

MY JOURNEY
FAMILY CHAOS

For months, life inside the walls of our home had been anything but normal. We all might have looked fine, but we were not fine at all. Our lives had been turned upside down with the stress of the cancer diagnosis and treatment.

BREAST CANCER IMPACTS EVERYONE

I remember one morning, between my biopsies, when my mom was still visiting, that things just fell apart. Dan and I got into a disagreement about school that quickly escalated into chaos. After just a few moments, I was crying, Dan was yelling, my mom was trying to find a graceful way to escape upstairs, and Dave was somehow trying to finish up a conference call. Ken looked over at the drama from his computer and tried to find a way not to get involved. After months of family stress that started with my diagnosis process, we were all well beyond the breaking point. It didn't take much to set us off into a family fight.

Most of the time, these incidents were an explosion of the stress and fears we were all having. The entire family dynamic had shifted for us. We love our routines, and this didn't look like anything we had experienced before. Dave was cooking dinners and I was recuperating upstairs. The kids needed help with their school, but I was unavailable. Emotions were running high.

One of the ways that we tried to address and acknowledge the challenge of cancer was to communicate openly with each other. Dave ended up taking the lead on this because I was not in any emotional shape to talk it out while I was recovering. He would have the boys join him for a dog walk. While they were busy tiring the beagles, he would let them vent and express themselves.

CANCER & THE KIDS

I chose to be open with my kids about my cancer diagnosis and treatment. Since they were both teenage boys, there were a few times that the conversation ended in embarrassed giggles because we were talking about breasts at the dinner table.

The boys and I were talking at the dinner table recently about my treatment and how things were going now. Dan said to me, "It wasn't easy, but I learned a lot. I learned how to plan ahead for my school and do the assignments on my own without Mom's help. I had two choices: do it myself, or work with Dad. Since working with Dad usually meant the work took longer, it was easier to do it myself. I learned how to be more independent."

Ken shared, "I really didn't think about your cancer treatment while it was going on. I buried a lot of my emotions. I wanted to become the pillar of support that you could lean on when things were difficult. In the end, I never came to grasp what emotions I had about the cancer. By letting my feelings fester, I erupted in grief periodically after the treatment was over. All the emotions came up for me once it was all done. I probably should have talked about it more while it was happening."

It wasn't an easy time for my kids, and I often wonder how their lives will be shaped long-term. I'm grateful for their support, but there are times I grieve for the fun we didn't get to have during my treatment.

I watched my sons cope with my mortality in very different ways. As I mentioned before, Ken was quiet and processed his emotions by himself. If he was feeling angry or frustrated, it wasn't visible to me. I missed a lot of his activities, but he would always come and give me an update on how his baseball practice went, or what the latest work adventure was. He would show his love in practical acts of service. If I needed anything, like a water bottle or a heating pad, he would drop what he was doing and bring it to me.

Dan wanted to talk everything out. I knew exactly what he was feeling because he didn't hide anything. There were quite a few tearful moments while he shared how terrified he was that I might die. He had never thought about me dying before, and cancer was scary. I also noticed that he was often angry during my treatment and recovery. His foundation and routine had been shaken, and it was frightening. It was hard to watch him struggle, but I also began to realize how deeply he loved me. The negative emotions were a reaction to his fear of losing me. As I listened, sat with him, hugged him, and spent time with him, I found that our relationship took on a new depth and sweetness.

As I began my recovery and transitioned back into my usual role, we had some significant power struggles. Dad had been in charge for months while I had focused on healing. Now I was back in charge and doing things differently. In some ways, the kids were glad that I was back to add some more flexibility to the discipline. While I had resumed my usual duties, I was most definitely not back to full strength. There were many days I was grouchy, tired, and emotional.

THE RECOVERY PROCESS
WE DON'T BOUNCE BACK RIGHT AWAY

I wanted to jump right back into my life after treatment, but my body had other ideas. I would get winded easily on walks and get exhausted after doing the dishes. I needed to be patient and kind with myself as I approached my physical well-being. I needed to ask for help and be aware of what my limitations were.

At the beginning of my recovery, I made it my goal to try to get through the day without feeling completely exhausted. If I was grouchy or fatigued by dinner time, I had tried to do too much. I needed to modify my schedule and put in rest periods so that I could make it through the entire day.

Surgery and treatment are taxing on our physical well-being. We may have had months of treatment and restrictions on our exercise. We might need physical therapy to regain our strength and mobility. Additionally, if we are having reconstruction, there may be multiple surgeries yet to go. This can be frustrating because we want to get back to our "normal" as soon as possible so that we can feel recovered.

I prefer to think of recovery as an active process rather than an event. I'm not going to wake up one day feeling completely recovered. The scars and memories will always be there. But, if I think about it as a process that I'm working through, I feel less frustrated. It will take time to rebuild stamina after treatment.

OTHERS' JOURNEYS
RETURNING TO WORK

During my interviews with other breast cancer survivors, I asked how they handled their work during treatment and recovery. I share some of their stories here so that you can see how others approached their time off and return to work.

davita Had just started a new job right before her breast cancer diagnosis. She ended up working through some parts of her chemotherapy. "I went back to work during chemo but waited until I was just on the Taxol [a chemotherapy drug that can be better tolerated than others]. I went back to work on number five of eight rounds. I took it easy and listened to my body. I was upfront with my teams and told them what was going on and everyone was caring."[2]

noelle Also took time off of work during her surgery and recovery. "I was lucky to be able to take off work during my treatment, surgery, and recovery. I was lucky to be able to receive California state disability along with some other financial assistance from some amazing non-profits. I work for Southwest Airlines, and they were incredibly supportive when I left for medical leave as well as when I returned. The love and support I received from my work group and leaders was amazing."[3]

jill A student at the time of her diagnosis. "Personally, I would not have been able to work during chemotherapy because my side effects were so severe. I am very thankful that I was not working at the time. For those who are, be open and honest about your treatment with your employer, talk with your doctors about time off, if needed, and never stop advocating for yourself for what you need."[4]

jennifer f. Worked up until surgery, but then needed to go on disability because her treatment plan changed. "My plan changed, and I was being referred for chemotherapy and radiation. I ended up being out of work for six months. While I struggled with guilt for not powering through and balancing work and home with my treatments (like many women can do), I am glad I took that time off to focus on my health. Once I returned to work, I felt ready and energized. I am better prepared to keep that balance in a healthy way because, in the end, maintaining my health is my number one goal."[5]

HOW DID I REINTEGRATE AFTER ACTIVE TREATMENT?

Returning to our daily work routines can be a welcome aspect of our recovery. As we add things back into our lives, it is possible that we begin to feel the emotional toll that breast cancer has taken on us.

Once my treatment ended, I tried to return gradually to my daily routines. Dave had time off for Christmas. It was great to have him off work and helping out while I dealt with the residual fatigue. He returned to work and travel after the New Year. During that first month, I was still limiting my activities to minimize my exhaustion. It was quite challenging to run the household again, especially when he was out of town.

Another part of my recovery was learning how to have fun again. I finally had the energy to hang out with the kids, and we would laugh at TV shows and play games together. I remember Dan looking at me and saying, "I missed hearing you laugh." I didn't realize that we had stopped having fun together while I was in treatment, perhaps because I was just too fatigued to notice.

UNWELCOME EMOTIONS
GUILT & MOOD SWINGS

It was hard for me not to get sucked into a guilt spiral. My cancer diagnosis had impacted everyone in the family.

The kids were doing more chores; Dave was taking time away from work; we weren't able to see our family and friends. It was tough.

One of the most emotional decisions that we made was to cancel our post-Christmas trip to see Dave's parents. They had moved to Idaho a few years before, and we were going to celebrate the dawn of 2020 with them. We decided to cancel because we were unsure how I would be doing after finishing treatment. I was concerned about potential side effects that I might have and how hard it would be to get back to my doctors if I needed to.

I had a lot of guilt about that decision. I wanted so much to be able to push through the treatment and have the strength to do the trip. But radiation was wiping me out and I could barely make it through the day. I would be much more comfortable recovering at home, in my own space.

This guilt wasn't productive. If I stayed in that emotional space, I wouldn't be able to make progress with my emotional recovery. I spent a lot of time talking to Dave. He was a great listener and helped me untangle some of the challenging feelings.

One of the ways that I tried to deal with the feeling of guilt was to change the way I was thinking about my day-to-day decisions. When I was saying "no" to something that would exhaust me, I was making an active choice to say "yes" to my recovery. This was a way for me to reframe the guilt into something productive. Every time I chose rest over stress, I was helping my body and soul rebuild.

For years, I had drifted into a pattern of taking care of everyone else's needs first. I wanted all of the people in my life to be happy, and *then* I could be happy. This was an unrealistic and unhealthy perspective. I allowed my happiness and contentment to be tied with the emotions of others.

The cancer wasn't making any of us happy, and there wasn't anything I could do to make it better. I needed to break out of that codependent strategy and become aware of my real feelings. I needed more emotional ownership in my life. Making the choice to break out of the guilt spiral was a way I could move forward.

It wasn't easy, especially since I started taking tamoxifen just a few weeks after finishing radiation. I was short-tempered, irritable, and still exhausted. I yelled a lot that first month I was on the tamoxifen. In fact, I got some commentary from the boys that the drug was "making me crazy." Just the mention of how the tamoxifen impacted me would often set me into a rage, reinforcing the "crazy mom" imagery.

After a few of those comments, we all sat down at the dinner table and had a family discussion. I told the boys why I was taking the pill and explained that it was hard on me, but I wanted to try it so that I would reduce the risk of getting cancer again. I told them that they weren't allowed to tell me that the medicine was "making me crazy." Dave told them that commenting on my medicine was off limits. If the boys needed to talk about their feelings, he was willing to take them on a walk. I was in no shape to deal with those conversations.

I appreciated that he was reinforcing boundaries in the home to help protect my well-being. If you are interested in learning more about how to establish effective boundaries for yourself, I highly recommend that you read *Set*

Boundaries, Find Peace: A Guide to Reclaiming Yourself, by Nedra Glover Tawwab. It is an extremely practical book and has been a help to me as I navigate my limits after cancer treatment.

When I felt my emotions get so heated that I wasn't able to communicate calmly, I would walk away. I went up to my room, put on some calming music, and tried to center myself. I would pray, meditate, or just breathe. When I felt myself calming down, I would go back to the situation and see if I was able to re-engage without the heightened emotions. After a month or so, I wasn't feeling the emotional effects of the tamoxifen quite as much, and I was better able to acknowledge my feelings without having a conversation that progressed to a yell-fest.

MENTAL WELL-BEING
UNEXPECTED BRAIN FOG

I eagerly anticipated returning to my French classes once I completed treatment. I thought I would have a small dip in my progress, but I didn't expect how difficult it would be to read aloud and access the French words for conversation. It was as if I was swimming through cognitive mud. There were a few times I had absolutely no idea what word I was looking for in the middle of a discussion. This was more than just missing a couple of weeks of classes. Before my diagnosis and treatment, I had been studying intently for a French fluency exam. I was speaking and comprehending better than I ever had before. Now, I was struggling to reach for the right words. What was going on?

This brain fog was very unsettling. I found that I had less attention and thinking power during and just after active treatment. I knew that chemotherapy could have an impact on our brains, but I hadn't had chemo. What was going on?

My first target was stress. I had been taxed mentally for months, and the stress was an obvious culprit. I kept doing research, and I was shocked to find out new research links endocrine therapies, such as tamoxifen, with cognitive decline similar to that of chemotherapy.[6] *Cognitive decline* or *impairment* is the medical term used to describe the loss of our intelligence and thinking power. I was angry when I read about this side effect. I knew to expect the mood swings and the vaginal dryness, but now I learned I was taking a drug that could impact my intelligence. Research is still being done on this aspect of endocrine therapy, and I hope that oncologists will include this possible side effect in their discussions with patients.

I decided to take an active role in attacking the brain fog. I began to gradually increase my cognitive challenges. I began writing this book shortly after finishing radiation treatment. I set aside time each day for reading. At first, I only had energy for short bursts of reading, but the more I read, the easier it got. I also made time each day to listen to, read, and practice my French. Returning to the weekly classes gave me the incentive I needed to challenge myself and try to get back to the level I had achieved before treatment.

After a few months, I was able to converse more freely in class again. The fog had begun to lift. I felt encouraged that the small steps I was taking to challenge myself were making a difference.

If you are experiencing fuzziness and brain fog after treatment, you are not alone. Breast cancer treatment is stressful, and that has an impact on our ability to think clearly. Also, the chemo or medications have an impact on our brains. I encourage you to discuss challenges with your medical team and approach this recovery process with patience.

EMOTIONAL WELL-BEING
ACKNOWLEDGING THE FEARS OF RECURRENCE

I was making great progress with my physical recovery and feeling more mentally strong as Spring 2020 continued. Things were going well, until my anxiety decided to return. I began to experience fears of recurrence as my imaging appointments approached.

As I faced the MRI and mammogram for my six-month imaging, I got really anxious. My MRI had been troublesome before. What were they going to find? I found myself spinning in anxiety as I approached these scans. No imaging had been done after my lumpectomy or radiation. I wondered if they had gotten all the cancer.

It turns out this fear has a special name. It is called "scanxiety." It wasn't pleasant to experience at all. I've tried to manage my fears of recurrence by enjoying the six months I have in between imaging appointments; They aren't looking for breast cancer in me every week, so it doesn't do me any good to worry about a recurrence in between my scans. I had a few years of clear imaging, and then, I didn't.

In June of 2022, about two and a half years after my DCIS diagnosis, I had another breast cancer scare. Imaging revealed a finding on my left breast, the non-cancer side, that had increased in size significantly. The following months were full of anxiety as I dealt with the possibility that I might have cancer again. You can read more about my experiences in Summer 2022 in the epilogue, but I'm thrilled to share that this time, it wasn't cancer!

I would not be surprised if I have another breast cancer event, or another scare, in the future. My cancer was estrogen receptor-positive. My body is still producing estrogen, and I wasn't able to continue with the tamoxifen. Since I am continuing with my imaging as directed, the doctors are able to document and take action on any changes they discover, as they did in Summer 2022. Acknowledging the possibility of a recurrence helps me move forward with my life and gives me a sense of urgency. I can't wait for the right time to do things that are important to me—now is that time.

13
SEX. YES, SEX
(or lack thereof)

DAVE AND I HAD just returned from a couple's trip to the Caribbean when my diagnosis process kicked into high gear. Our tropical vacation had been a time to talk, have fun, and prioritize the sexy side of our relationship. I had skimpy bikinis and stylish coverups that I would wear during the day, then I would change into a dress at night for dinner and dancing. I felt beautiful and sexy.

When we returned, the biopsies began. Not only did they take pieces of my breast tissue out, but they also seemed to remove my sex drive! I was stressed, in pain, and worried, and I had bruises on my breasts. My breasts, which had been clothed in a sequined bikini just a few weeks before, were now being poked, prodded, and examined by my new medical team. The glow of intimacy I felt after the vacation evaporated, and I wasn't sure if it would ever return.

For nearly three months, Dave was my caregiver. When my treatment finished, we could focus on rebuilding our partnership. Intimacy had taken a backseat to cancer for the last several months. I wondered if it would recover, or if the damage was permanent.

ACKNOWLEDGING OUR UNIQUE SITUATIONS

As I delve into my sexuality and experiences, I want to acknowledge that my situation may look very different from yours. I hope that this window into my sexuality as a breast cancer survivor can help you see and find clarity no matter what your relationship status or sexual orientation. Reclaiming our sexuality after cancer is challenging whether we are single, married, divorced, partnered, or widowed. As you navigate these waters, I encourage you to seek out support that will enable you to build a fulfilling intimate life.

MY JOURNEY
BREASTS WERE NO LONGER SYMBOLS OF MY FEMININITY

Before my breast cancer diagnosis, I had been enjoying some creativity with my daily lingerie choices. I had purchased some beautiful lacy bras on our trips to France, and I enjoyed wearing them each day. I would pair them with pretty lace panties to complete the look. Getting dressed each morning was a private ritual for me to acknowledge and embrace my femininity. I felt beautiful in my French bras.

I couldn't wear these bras after my first biopsy. The underwire of my beautiful bras pressed against the biopsy area and hurt too much. Instead, when I got dressed in the morning, I would pick out which sports bra would work with my top of the day. I would look longingly at my pretty bras every morning, and even try to wear them occasionally. After a few minutes of pain, I would take them off in disappointment and put the sports bra back on. Eventually, I took the French bras out of my drawer and placed them in a basket on a high shelf in my closet. Perhaps, one day, I would be able to wear them again.

It didn't help that during every appointment I was showing my breasts to my doctors. They stopped being symbols of my femininity. In many ways, my breasts didn't feel like they were mine anymore. When Dave would touch them during our intimacy, I would have flashbacks of the latest medical procedure.

Dealing with those memory flashes was really disturbing. In retrospect, I could have chosen to stop and talk to Dave about it as it was happening, but I was so disoriented that I just tried to block it out and detach. That didn't help me enjoy the touching, either. I would go through the motions of intimacy, but my mind was somewhere else.

After my lumpectomy and radiation, I had hoped things would get back to normal, but I was still dealing with residual pain and uncomfortable memories. Over the course of several months, the flashbacks began to subside.

When I felt a flashback coming, I tried to pay close attention to the sensory details going on to stay in the moment. I would listen to the music, look at the soft lighting, notice the expression on my husband's face, and try to pay attention to what the touching felt like. I also would redirect the touching to other areas if I was having trouble staying present.

I was really frustrated about this situation. I had made a deliberate choice to keep my breasts with a lumpectomy and now I didn't want anyone to touch them. Things were complicated for me, and for Dave.

I watched Dave struggle with emotions and uncertainty. He wasn't sure if he could touch my breasts, didn't know what things would be like after treatment, and feared a potential future without me.

While these emotions would come up for us during lovemaking, it often wasn't the best time to talk about them. I struggled to put my feelings into words while in the moment. It was much easier for me to talk about my sexual fears and challenges when we were out walking. The rhythmic pace helped unlock my words, and being outside made it easier for me to keep my emotions in check. It was hard to talk about how breast cancer impacted our sex life. This was a dynamic and enjoyable part of our relationship that was suddenly on life support.

CHALLENGES OF ENJOYING SEX DURING TREATMENT

While I didn't want to stop having sex during the months I was in breast cancer treatment, the frequency and quality of our intimacy was impacted. Whether it was pain, exhaustion, or difficulty in positioning, sex had become more like a complicated puzzle than an enjoyable time together.

I was very sore after my five biopsies, surgery, and radiation. I had hoped that once the skin stopped peeling, my sensation would return to normal, but the tissue inside my right breast was still painful from the radiation treatment. It took months for my insides to feel recovered.

After my surgery, one of the instructions that my surgeon gave me was to not "bounce my breasts" or squish them. Sex typically involves a certain amount of breast bouncing, so I needed to get creative. One of the things I did was wear a bra during lovemaking to keep them in place.

We also needed to be flexible in our positioning. I discovered that being on my knees was the most comfortable position. This allowed me to stay in one position and not bounce. It also kept my breasts out of center stage when I was uncomfortable about their appearance. I also found this position comfortable during radiation when my skin was sensitive.

When I wasn't feeling self-conscious about how my breasts looked, being on top worked well. This position kept my breasts from being squished but was better suited for me when I was more recovered from surgery because I moved more when I was on top.

All this positioning and pain impacted my enjoyment. I had very little sex drive at all during treatment. One of the pamphlets that I got before radiation said, "Sexual desire or performance may change during treatment." I showed this to Dave, and we laughed. That sentence was a huge understatement. I was exhausted, emotional, and in pain. Sex was more of an afterthought, if it happened at all.

I wasn't the only one struggling with sexual desire. Earlier, in chapter 9, I shared that I had attempted to boost Dave's morale with a passionate kiss, only to have him pull away. After a good cry, I worked up the courage to talk about it with him. He opened up and shared that he, too, was dealing with a lower sex drive. He was expending a lot of energy taking care of the household, the virtual schooling, my care needs, and the meal preparation. At the end of the day, we were both feeling exhausted and drained. Lovemaking wasn't something for which we had much energy.

I wondered if things would recover after treatment. Would we get back to the place we were after our Caribbean vacation? I was afraid as to what our intimate relationship would look like after cancer. I wasn't ready to say goodbye to that part of myself, but I didn't know what the future would look like for us.

NO SEXUAL BOUNCE-BACK AFTER TREATMENT

My fears were more than just about the mechanics of our sexual life. Over the years, the quality of our lovemaking has been a barometer for our intimate partnership. When my husband and I are connected, working together well, and enjoying one another, our lovemaking reflects that oneness.

It wasn't a big surprise that it was hard to enjoy one another sexually while I was in active treatment, but I hoped that our sex life would recover, both in frequency and in passion, once I finished radiation.

It turns out that we would have other challenges to face. While I was in treatment, Dave and I were both looking forward to spending our twentieth anniversary together in France. That trip, which would be about four months after I finished radiation, would be our finish line. We would enjoy time away, just the two of us, and have the time to figure out what our sexual relationship looked like after cancer.

That trip was planned for April 2020. As COVID-19 began to spread, we realized that this finish line was in danger. A few weeks before the trip, everything shut down. If we were going to sort out our sexuality, it wouldn't be on a lovely vacation, it would be during a year of staying home.

It took a while for us to really get our sex life sorted out after treatment. The after effects of treatment were physical, mental, and emotional. I could use lubricant to make it comfortable, but was I able to enjoy the time with my partner? I was physically present, but there were times my mental and emotional presence were elsewhere.

Sexual challenges are not uncommon during and after breast cancer. I'll share some of the common issues that survivors face, but this isn't a comprehensive list. This is a complicated area, and I highly recommend that you seek out professional support if you and your partner are struggling with this aspect of your relationship.

Lingering Breast Pain. I had pain inside my radiated breast for months after treatment. Once the skin finished peeling, I gave Dave the green light to touch my right breast again. That was short lived because it was still painful deep inside. The radiation had reached into the breast tissue, and it was sore for nearly four months.

Discomfort with Taking Pleasure from Breast Stimulation. I still have sensation in my breasts and nipples because I chose a lumpectomy. In fact, preserving sensation was one of the biggest reasons that I decided to do this surgery. But I have a real mental challenge now about receiving pleasure from breast stimulation. We would be in the middle of lovemaking, and I would flash back to a medical appointment. Since so many of my treatments were on my breast, sometimes all it would take would be the touch on my breast to trigger a memory. This is an ongoing challenge, even a few years after treatment.

Numbness. If you have had mastectomy, your reconstructed breasts may be numb. This may also be the case if you choose to go without reconstruction. Numbness may be something that you and your partner need to adapt to during your intimacy.

Uncomfortable with New Appearance. I was shocked at how bruised I was after my lumpectomy. I was also a little frustrated with the location of one of my scars. Every time I showered, I would wonder if I should have left that benign lump in so that I wouldn't have the scar in such a noticeable place. Physical scars are a reality of this cancer treatment journey. As I was applying lotion to my breasts during radiation, I tried to pay attention to my "mental talk" as I cared for my skin. If I was frustrated at the appearance, I would try to reframe it as thankfulness that the cancer had been removed. It took months for me to really feel comfortable with my scars and accept them.

Sexual Desire on Endocrine Treatment. The endocrine medications, such as tamoxifen and aromatase inhibitors, are not kind to sex drive. I noticed a marked decrease in my sexual desire as soon as I started the medicine. Medically induced menopause, due to medication, surgery, or treatments, can have a negative impact on sexual desire, even more than natural menopause.

Vaginal Dryness. Not only did I have trouble with desire, now intercourse and clitoral stimulation hurt! My vaginal walls dried out within weeks of starting the tamoxifen. It was so severe that I had to ask my gynocologist to run a test to make sure that I wasn't having an infection. I didn't have the mental desire to have sex, and now it hurt. I brought these concerns up with my doctor and, after she ruled out an infection, she gave me several ideas to try. She recommended OTC lubricants and vaginal moisturizers, and she also got clearance from my oncologist to prescribe low-dose vaginal estrogen. I ended up finding a lubricant that worked well and didn't irritate my skin.

Decreased Orgasmic Intensity. My orgasms were harder to achieve, and they were not as intense. My clitoral tissues were dry, which made the rubbing uncomfortable. Manual stimulation needed to be gentle so as not to irritate me. I appreciated oral sex because it added moisture to the area, but, even with the gentle stimulation, I found that my orgasms weren't as intense. I needed to put more mental focus into the process, which made it harder for me to let go. I was constantly worried that something was going to hurt or that I just wouldn't be able to have an orgasm. The worry was an unproductive companion during our lovemaking.

COMMUNICATE CLEARLY ABOUT YOUR COMFORT

One of the first things I tried to address in my sexuality after breast cancer was my own physical comfort. If things were hurting, I wouldn't enjoy it, and I wouldn't want to do it again.

I was up front with Dave about what was hurting. I also worked with my medical team to develop strategies to help me be comfortable during intercourse. If my vagina was raw, it was time to take a break and get more creative. There were a few times that I needed to take an extended rest from intercourse because it was too painful.

While I know that communication is important, I don't like talking during sex. If I try to have a conversation, my arousal level decreases. This made for some interesting challenges. I had to get over my hang up about talking during lovemaking to share what was working and what wasn't. It was hard, but worth it.

Here are a few ideas to consider as you think about your physical well-being during lovemaking:

Communicate what is working. If you like something, let your partner know. This positive feedback will enhance your pleasure and help your partner better understand your needs.

Communicate clearly what isn't working. If something is making you uncomfortable, feels painful, or just isn't working, say something. Your partner isn't feeling what you are and may not be aware that the friction is hurting you.

Identify what is pleasurable. In order for the intimate partnership to work well, it is essential to know what is pleasurable for you. This may take time and patience to figure out. It may be beneficial to spend time exploring touch and sensation on your own to see what hurts and what feels good. Once you are aware of what is working, then it is easier to communicate to your partner.

Choose positions carefully. After breast cancer, I discovered that certain positions were uncomfortable for me during lovemaking. I was uncomfortable with my breasts being on display as I was adjusting to my new appearance, so being on top wasn't a good choice. For a while, the missionary position was not possible because it would put pressure on my breasts. One of the most comfortable and pleasurable positions was to be on all fours. This allowed me to stay in one position, protected my breasts from bouncing, kept them out of center stage, and was the most pleasurable.

Be creative. Sexuality doesn't always need to mean intercourse. There may be other ways to experience sexual pleasure that are more enjoyable and comfortable after treatment. If you are feeling uncomfortable with your appearance, perhaps dimming the lights would enhance your comfort.

I tried to cultivate creativity and exploration during the months after treatment.

Be patient with pleasure. I took my ability to orgasm for granted before breast cancer. During and after treatment, the anxiety, pain, hormonal changes, and medical flashbacks made it difficult to have an orgasm. I wondered at times if our sex life would be one-sided. Would breast cancer take away my ability to enjoy intimacy? I feared that this would be permanent. The more I focused on whether I could orgasm, the less I was able to. It was a very unfulfilling cycle. Some of these challenges were physical and could be addressed with communication and positioning. But there were also mental and emotional issues that I needed to work through that impacted my ability to enjoy intimacy.

OTHERS' JOURNEYS
SEX: A DIFFICULT TOPIC TO DISCUSS

It was challenging to find people willing to talk about this topic. In fact, when I posted about this on Twitter, I got a fantastic response about the topic from Mia: "The elephant in the room of #breastcancer SEX."[1] The following are responses that I got from a very lively Twitter conversation on the topic.

kate "I found, while on chemo, I was too tired. So instead we have massaged each other. Sometimes that ended in sex. But it was nice to be touched and still feel attractive, even when I felt horrible. Talking helps too. There's nothing more intimate than that."[2]

flori "I've learned that sex and feeling sexy is so much more than individual body parts. Lingerie became a dear friend. Made me feel like me in the beginning. Helped my self-esteem until I was more used to my scars and new parts."[3]

jody "I was 43 and kept my breasts following bi-lateral diagnosis. Dual lumpectomies and radiation. Intimacy was a big part of that decision. Condoms during chemo and other fun as well like all the hair loss. Hubs loved the bald below the belt."[4]

she "Scream Cream* . . . a little dab will do ya! (*RX compound topical that puts the OHHHH back in orgasm). Ladies, cancer meds often affect our libidos. Solutions for many of our issues are out there. Talk to a cancer friend [and/or] be creative—go look for them. Bring your sexy back!"[5]

MENTAL WELL-BEING
ACCEPTANCE

It wasn't enough for me to address the physical challenges of sexuality after breast cancer. I needed to deal with the thoughts in my head during intimacy.

The first thing that helped me was to remove the judgment I was placing on myself. If my thoughts wandered to a medical flashback, I could gently steer myself back to the moment. I didn't need to judge myself for those thoughts. Being gentle, kind, and accepting of the mental chatter helped me enjoy the intimacy. I acknowledged it was there and could then choose to refocus my thoughts. I would concentrate on the sensations, listen to the music in the background, and notice my partner's enjoyment. Gradually, I found myself becoming more present and aware.

I also gave myself permission not to have sexual desire. This may seem like a strange statement. Why would I need to give myself permission, and how would that help? Before breast cancer, I had become comfortable with the ebbs and flows of my sexual desire. I knew that there were certain times of the month when I especially enjoyed lovemaking. I would be more engaged, and my orgasms would be more intense. I also knew that right before my period, my desire would plummet.

Tamoxifen seemed to put my sexual desire on idle. It didn't matter what time of the month it was, I just wasn't interested. I could get frustrated about that, but I wouldn't be able to make progress and move forward. I decided to accept my state of reduced desire. I still wanted to be comfortable and have pleasure during intimacy, but I would be more accepting of where I was. Guilt trips were not going to help me get aroused faster.

I didn't become fully aware of how low my desire had been until I went off of tamoxifen, at the direction of my oncologist. I look back on the months I was on tamoxifen, and I am shocked at how much it impacted my desire, sexual comfort, and orgasm quality. Within a month of going off the drug, I was enjoying intimacy again. It was more than just my vaginal tissues regaining moisture;

I was able to experience pleasure at a deeper level. My orgasms were more satisfying, and my sex drive returned.

EMOTIONAL WELL-BEING
TALKING THROUGH FRUSTRATING FEELINGS

I was frustrated with all the sexual issues I faced after breast cancer. In an appointment with my gynecologist, I was honest with her that I wasn't willing to stay on a drug that killed my sexuality. I was 42 and in a vibrant and passionate marriage. I was not willing to say goodbye to the sexual side of myself.

She was so supportive. She told me she wanted all her patients to have the ability to enjoy as much sex as they wanted. She was willing to work with me, listen to my issues, and give me detailed suggestions. I felt validated after that appointment. She was the first doctor I ever had who viewed my sexuality and pleasure as an integral component of my personhood. I've had conversations with doctors in the past about pain during intercourse, and they've brushed me off. Not this doctor. She listened and cared. Her support helped me feel less frustrated about my emotions.

If you are feeling frustrated, I would recommend you find someone to whom you can talk. This person may be your partner. It could also be a trusted friend or a medical professional. I have also found much support in breast cancer groups. Sometimes a listening ear can help us work through these difficult emotions.

Along with frustration, I also felt sad. I had kept my breasts, but they weren't bringing me much enjoyment during intimacy. They still hurt, I was uncomfortable with my scars, and I had medical flashbacks during lovemaking. I was unhappy that my orgasms weren't satisfying and that I had to work so hard to stay in the moment.

I was devastated that Dave and I weren't able to celebrate our wedding anniversary in France and that we had no romantic dates to look forward to. Everything we had done in the past to reconnect emotionally and cultivate our sexual relationship was turned upside down with the pandemic. How were we going to be vital and passionate with teenagers in the home all of the time?

BUILDING INTIMACY OUTSIDE THE BEDROOM

For the most intimate parts of our relationship to function well, Dave and I needed to find a way to cultivate it. This was challenging because we didn't have the privacy we were accustomed to. The entire family was home all the time during the pandemic. We needed to find a pandemic-friendly way to work through our intimacy challenges and reconnect on a romantic level.

One of the ways that Dave and I did that was through long walks. We would go out for about an hour and a half on weekend mornings and walk the trails near our home. This provided us with some privacy so that we could talk about our sex life out of earshot of the kids. It was easier for me to talk about my struggles when I wasn't in the moment. The walking seemed to allow my thoughts to flow into words.

LOOKING AHEAD TO THE FUTURE

As the months passed from my treatment, I discovered that I was able to talk about the future again. While I was in treatment, Dave would want to talk about his hopes and dreams. I was not willing to look that far ahead. I simply couldn't predict that I would ever feel well again. He wanted to dream, and I was just trying to get through to the next day.

It was progress when I realized I could talk with Dave about our dreams again. Sharing those conversations with him helped us deepen our intimacy and partnership. Our children will be grown in just a few years. There is change coming in our marriage, and I'm thankful that I can hope again.

These hopes were not just for my marriage, they were also dreams of what I might do after my days as a virtual school parent were over. I only had a few years left of this role. What did I want to do with the next chapter of my life? I began to sense that this DCIS diagnosis was not going to be something I would walk through and move on from. I felt a new sense of purpose. I felt a passion and mission to share my story and help others along the way. There was a transformation happening inside me as I walked through my recovery.

14
FINDING A NEW BEAUTIFUL
getting to know the post-cancer you

AS I BEGAN TO feel a mental transformation, there were lingering reminders of treatment I couldn't ignore. I walked out of radiation treatment with my right breast inflamed and incredibly sunburned. My treatment was completed, but my body hadn't recovered from the trauma. It would be a few weeks until the peeling finished and months until the soreness resolved. My left breast, which hadn't had the radiation, was now visibly smaller than the right. I had always been slightly lopsided, but now it seemed more noticeable.

I was finished with my active treatment, but my body was still healing. People would comment on how good I looked, and I would laugh because they couldn't see the purple burns on my breast from radiation. I was exhausted and didn't know when I would get my energy back. I was still adjusting to the tamoxifen, so I had mood swings to deal with and hot flashes that would come out of nowhere.

Once my treatment ended, the recovery process became much more private. I wrote my support team one final note once my radiation was finished, and then I stopped with the updates. It was time to walk the recovery journey within.

MY JOURNEY
REDEFINING MY PERSONAL STYLE

It was a few weeks after my surgery, and I was getting ready for church. I pulled a dress over my head and asked Dave to zip me up. This vintage floral dress was one of my favorites, and I loved to wear it. Then I looked in the mirror. Who was this person staring back at me? Something wasn't right.

I unzipped the dress, put it back on the hanger, and picked another one. That one didn't work either. These beautiful, vintage-style dresses seemed all wrong. What was going on?

Some Sunday mornings it would take four tries for me to find something that worked. I was so frustrated. I kept apologizing to Dave because it was taking forever for me to get ready. He said, "You're going through identity trauma during this treatment. It's okay. Take your time."

Those floral dresses, which had been my signature church dresses, now felt like they belonged to the woman I was before cancer. There was transformation and transition going on in my mindset and my sense of personal identity. I went back to my closet, found a simple black dress, and paired it with a scarf. As I looked in the mirror once again, I smiled. I was beginning to dress as the woman I was becoming.

HOW DO WE FEEL & LOOK AFTER TREATMENT?

The challenges I had with putting on dresses for church were one small indication that I had more growth ahead of me. It would take time to address all of the components of my well-being after active treatment. While your recovery might not involve redefining your wardrobe, like mine did, it will take time. Recovery isn't an event that occurs, it is a process we walk through.

HEALING, ADJUSTING & REGAINING STRENGTH

Our physical healing from cancer treatment takes time. There may be lingering side effects from treatment such as fatigue, skin peeling, hair loss, and neuropathy. In some cases, time will resolve these issues. With other side effects, there may be additional treatments and physical therapy needed to address the issues.

> **Fatigue.** I felt my fatigue begin to lift a few weeks after completing radiation treatment. I first noticed it when I didn't need to go to bed as early each night. I still got tired during the day, but I didn't need as much sleep as I did during treatment. Cancer treatment and surgery takes a lot out of our bodies, and they need time to rebuild. I recommend gradually adding activities back in and removing things if you find yourself getting too exhausted at the end of the day.
>
> **Skin Peeling.** My skin continued to darken and peel after my radiation treatment was completed. It was the most uncomfortable phase for me because I

was the most tender, and I just wanted to be done! I needed to be diligent about my lotions and my care for the skin as it recovered from the radiation treatment. A few months after treatment, my skin began to itch again. I didn't have any visible issues, but it was uncomfortable. I began putting lotion on again, and that helped the itchiness resolve.

Hair Regrowth. If you have had chemotherapy, your hair will likely begin to regrow once your treatment completes. Some women find that their hair grows back a different texture or color. Learning how to style your new, short hair and deal with the in-between phases can be a challenge. Davita has been experimenting with different styles and accessories as her hair has grown out. It doesn't grow back as quickly as it fell out, so this can be a long-term reminder of treatment. I recommend reaching out to your hairstylist as your hair begins to return and getting some recommendations. Getting the support of a professional may help you learn and embrace this in-between phase.

Neuropathy. Another side effect of chemotherapy is neuropathy, or nerve damage in your extremities. This condition can impact balance and fine motor control. If you are experiencing neuropathy, I would recommend discussing options with your medical team. There are some activities such as stretching, yoga, walking, and strength training that can be helpful to reduce the symptoms.

Lymphedema. If you have had lymph nodes removed or have had radiation treatment, you may develop lymphedema.[1] Symptoms can include swelling, aching, tingling, and discomfort in the arms. There are many ways to keep this condition under control, such as physical therapy, compression garments, and exercises. It is important to keep an eye out for symptoms and get them addressed promptly so that there isn't any permanent damage. The lymph fluid needs to move throughout the body, and when lymphedema occurs, it means that the fluid is stuck and not circulating.

Reconstruction and Fills. If you have had a mastectomy and are undergoing reconstruction, this is a process that may take several months. If you have had expanders placed, they will be filled in the office a number of times until the desired size has been achieved. Enlarging the expanders needs to be done over a period of time because the skin, and sometimes the muscles, need to be expanded gently. As the expanders get fuller, they can get heavy and uncomfortable. Once the expanders have been filled, another surgery will be performed to trade out the expanders for implants. Multiple procedures can slow the physical recovery down. Be patient with yourself as you complete this reconstruction process. While we may want to be done with it all at once, a gradual process is easier for our bodies to tolerate and can result in fewer complications.

Movement Challenges. If you have ever broken a bone or sprained an ankle, it is common to be sent to physical therapy after the injury. However, a physical therapy referral is not standard practice after breast cancer surgery. I think it should be because many women have issues with muscle weakness, range of motion, and shoulder pain after surgery. The tendency to hold still to keep the area safe for healing can actually lead to more pain and reduced range of motion. It is possible to get a referral to physical therapy by talking with your medical team.

After my lumpectomy, I began doing gentle stretches just a few days after surgery to protect my shoulders and arms from these issues. I was gentle, but also very deliberate. I had suffered from shoulder impingement just a few years before and didn't want to go through that again. I recommend talking to your medical team about safe exercises to do so that you can rebuild your strength and maintain your range of motion. Physical therapy can be highly effective if you are struggling.

Cording. As I mentioned before, another issue that can develop after breast cancer surgery is muscle cording, rope-like cords that are usually found on the under part of your arm. Muscle cording is common if a sentinel node biopsy has been done. Treatment for cording is a combination of physical therapy and massage. If you develop cording in your months of recovery, I recommend reaching out to your medical team for a treatment plan.

Physical Stamina. My stamina for exercise and everyday life didn't come back all at once. I needed to slowly add things back in so that I didn't feel exhausted. As you resume your everyday activities and return to work, keep an eye on how you feel at the end of the day. If you are exhausted, try to do a little less the next day. One of the ways that I tried to rebuild my physical stamina was to look at my daily habits and see if I could make any changes that would add to my energy level.

LIFESTYLE CHANGES

The end of active treatment can be an ideal time to look at changes we can make to enhance our physical well-being. I wasn't ready to tackle these issues while I was in treatment, but once I finished with radiation, I had the desire to rebuild my body and add in habits that would be beneficial to my physical health.

EATING

The first thing that I tried doing was to look at what I was eating every day. I haven't really paid much attention to my diet over the years. I have spent most of my time making sure that Dave had the right foods available for him. He lost nearly 200 pounds eleven years ago and has maintained a healthy weight since then with a variety of plans including exercise and diet. Most of my meal-planning energy has gone into making sure he has the right foods available.

When I got diagnosed with cancer, Dave decided to go plant-based. He discovered a variety of documentaries that espoused the benefits of eating less meat. These documentaries encouraged plant-based eating for cancer-risk reduction. Dave was struggling with my diagnosis and wanted to do something constructive. Changing his eating plan was something active he could do. He also felt better and more energized by eating this way.

I was not happy with this new eating plan! He had been following a low-fat, calorie-counting plan for years, and it made my meal planning easy. He could eat anything as long as he counted the calories. I was frustrated with this added complexity. Thankfully, he was willing to make me a steak anytime I wanted it.

Once I was done with active treatment, I felt more ready to change up my eating habits. I decided to try to eat more vegetables every day. I wasn't ready to give up meat as Dave had, but I knew that I didn't eat enough produce. I decided to make myself a salad each day for lunch.

Small changes can add up. I noticed that I felt more balanced. I didn't feel as tired after lunch. I also enjoy my midday meals much more. In the years since my treatment, I have since discovered some family-friendly, plant-based meals to add into our rotation.

EXERCISE

Another thing I decided to do for my physical well-being was to add in more strenuous exercise. Exercise can reduce the risk of a cancer recurrence.[2] Plus, exercise was something constructive I could do each day that would help me feel better.

A few months after I finished radiation, I decided to try some at-home fitness programs that had dance classes. I loved to dance as a child, so picking this activity again felt more like fun than working out.

It wasn't long before I noticed that I had much more energy throughout the day. This stamina was more than just the absence of the radiation fatigue. I was feeling more energetic than I had in years. I could stay awake until bedtime and didn't feel the need to collapse on the couch right after cooking dinner.

I was smiling more, as well. I loved dancing again. When I finished the workouts, I felt exhausted, but then that feeling would melt away and I would have a smile on my face and a skip in my step.

I look forward to my exercise time every morning. It helps me stay in shape and also improves my mindset each day. My thoughts are clearer after my workouts. It has been a great way to rebuild my body and my mind after the stress of treatment. It's also a good way for me to physically work out some of the anxiety I felt heading into my scans.

SCANXIETY
WILL THEY FIND SOMETHING NEW?

I don't know if my DCIS will return. Unfortunately, there is no treatment that can guarantee that I will not have a recurrence. I have many years left to live and have already had one instance of breast cancer. Recurrence is a possibility with any type of breast cancer. While my active treatment is completed for now, I am not in the clear for the rest of my life.

These fears come up for me as my regular scans approach. As I mentioned before, it is quite common for cancer survivors to experience scanxiety. Before my first follow-up MRI, I felt jumpy, fearful, and anxious. During my diagnosis, this scan had found several abnormalities, and I was fearful that this first post-treatment scan would result in additional biopsies. I did a lot of deep breathing and prayer as I faced this MRI. I was worried about what it would find, and I knew it would be days before I had the results. I couldn't bring anyone with me because of COVID-19 restrictions. It was frightening to go through the imaging again.

The phone rang a day after my MRI. When I heard my surgeon's voice, I was really nervous. "Jennifer, we have the results of your MRI. They are normal. I'll see you in the office after you have your next mammogram."

"Thank you so much for calling me," I replied in relief. The scanxiety melted away immediately. There weren't any MRI-guided biopsies in my near future.

One of the ways that I have chosen to deal with the anxiety of a recurrence is to live as fully as I can in between scans. Unless a palpable lump comes up, I won't have a cancer diagnosis in the six months or a year between my imagings. I have a choice to make: Will I live in fear and anxiety, or will I embrace the time I have between as an opportunity to enjoy my life?

Fear, anxiety, and worry are all common emotions to feel after treatment. We are well acquainted with cancer treatment and don't want to go through it again. If you discover that these thoughts are interfering with your daily life, I highly recommend seeking out psychological help. It is very common to have these types of issues after cancer and speaking to a therapist can help you develop strategies to address them and make progress in your survivorship.

OTHERS' JOURNEYS
POST-TREATMENT CHANGES

We will all walk along our recovery path differently. Finding our new beautiful means something unique to each of us. Here are a few ways that the women I interviewed found peace and joy with their post-treatment appearances.

dawn "After my double mastectomy, I had a very hard time identifying with myself sexually. I felt like Frankenstein every time I caught a reflection of myself, which made showering very tough as my glass shower stall was adjacent to the bathroom mirrors. I thought about getting nipples tattooed, but, in the end, I felt like that was just another lie (implants being lie #1) so I started looking at pictures of art tattooed on breasts on Pinterest and decided on a henna-looking design. Since I basically have 'zero' feeling on my chest, I arrived at the tattoo parlor thinking it was going to be a walk in the park—boy, was I wrong! In fact, there was so much pain that I never fully finished the cancer side, but I'm still absolutely thrilled with the outcome. The tattoos cover all my scars and now stand for something I chose vs the double mastectomy, which I had no choice in. I no longer feel like Frankenstein and am back to feeling like my normal self."[3]

janelle "After treatment, it was difficult to look at myself in the mirror because I didn't see the same woman. I looked physically different and felt emotionally different. As time went on, the silver linings of cancer began to present themselves in unusual ways. When my hair returned curly after chemo, I started getting many compliments from my friends, family, and even strangers. I have gotten more compliments on my hair in the last two years since treatment ended than I had in my entire life with straight hair. Cancer provided me the opportunity to change my look to a new beautiful."[4]

grace "For me, I lived with the philosophy of Kintsugi. I started to look at my body as a work of strength and art and stronger and more beautiful after each surgery. Having cancer isn't something to be ashamed of or hide from. Every day that we wake up to fight it, even after we're done with the initial battle, is worth celebrating. I do something every day to celebrate my 'win.' From having that little extra delicious treat, reading a trashy book or curling up for a midday nap, I look at every one of those as a celebration of my win and how much I love that I can still do those things."[5]

MENTAL WELL-BEING
NOW WHAT?

I stopped at the red light, eager to get home after picking a few things up at the store. I had this itchy feeling that I was forgetting something. I racked my brain for what I could have forgotten. I looked down at the clock and realized that it was 2:30, the time that I usually left for my radiation treatments. For a month, my daily routine had been scheduled around treatments.

The light turned green and I continued on my way home, marveling at the fact that I would no longer have my days broken up by radiation treatment. For months, I had scheduled my days around appointments, procedures, and treatment. I felt free and yet purposeless at the same time. The entire fall had been spent on cancer treatment. Now what?

I had stopped doing many of my activities during cancer treatment because I didn't have the energy or time for them. I realized that now I had the opportunity to selectively add things back in.

When our active treatment ends, there is an opportunity to evaluate our lives and see what will have a place in our post-cancer routine. Not every activity needs to return to our calendars after cancer treatment. Perhaps this is a time to try something new and leave out the things that didn't bring us joy.

I was excited to return to my French classes after treatment. That activity brought me joy and challenged me intellectually. I went back to classes a few months after finishing radiation. COVID-19 hit about a month later, so those classes turned into virtual sessions. Anything I had wanted to add back into my life needed to be done at home because of the pandemic. Thankfully, one of the dreams I was pursuing could be done at home.

I had always wanted to write a book. For years, I had been too scared to put my thoughts down on the page. What would people think of me if they read my words? It was easier to keep my ideas to myself. After breast cancer,

I was compelled to write my story down. If I could share encouragement with others facing a similar diagnosis, then somehow my pain and struggles would be worth it. This was a story I could write about.

Breast cancer could be an opportunity for you to pursue something you have always dreamed about. What has been holding you back?

I always thought that I had years ahead of me to write. I was willing to wait until the kids were grown and then begin writing. Breast cancer made me realize that my time on earth was limited. I don't know if I will have a recurrence, but I am no longer willing to wait for the perfect time to pursue my dreams. I will make the time now because I don't know what lies ahead.

EMOTIONAL WELL-BEING
NOT ALL PEACHY IN POST-CANCER LAND

In addition to the worries about recurrence and the anxiety about upcoming scans, I experienced other emotions after my active treatment ended. All throughout my treatment, I had felt loved and supported by my family, friends, and church. Once I finished radiation, that extra layer of support went away. It was not as if people stopped caring, but my treatment was done and there weren't any more updates to give. Everything just returned to normal. And, to add to that, the pandemic hit. I wasn't able to reconnect with my extended family and friends because I was taking extra precautions.

It was an emotional letdown. I still wanted to talk about how I was doing, but the urgency wasn't there. I ended up taking that need to process my treatment into my first draft of this book. Every morning, I would write for as long as I had energy for doing so. I started at the beginning and just expressed what happened. It was loosely told in a chronological manner, but there was no other formal structure.

The book you are reading today is not the draft I wrote right after finishing treatment. I look back and read it and feel those emotions of trauma and pain again. It was a raw expression of my treatment and told the story in detail. Writing helped me to process the emotions of trauma, fear, anger, loneliness, and frustration. It allowed me the privacy to explore how I wanted to think about breast cancer and figure out how I would frame the treatment in the big picture of my life.

Writing was a therapeutic process. The blank page always had time for me. It didn't judge me or tell me that I was making too much out of my DCIS. It was a place for me to express my fears. I didn't know if I would ever feel sexual and vibrant again. I could explore those thoughts safely and privately through my writing.

I have also found great support in reaching out and making friends with others in the cancer community. I wasn't active on social media during my treatment, so my support circle was a little more limited. I had friends who had been through breast cancer, but they were much older at the time of their diagnosis. Their treatments and concerns were different from mine. I'm now active in several groups and have found people who have had diagnoses similar to mine. I have found connection through video chats with other breast cancer patients.

As I process through my recovery, I am joining a much larger community of cancer survivors who share similar challenges. I feel supported when I share on Twitter that I'm having scanxiety. I don't feel as alone when I struggle with my scars.

Mixed in with the fears and negative emotions is also a renewed joy and appreciation for the everyday routines. I have an appreciation for my energy to get through the day.

When I stand at the stove cooking, I remember a time when I wasn't able to prepare dinner for my family. Cleaning and cooking had become a daily drudgery for me. I had done it for so many years, and I was weary. But after being unable to do the work during treatment, I learned some important lessons. The first was that I didn't need to do it all myself. My family could help me. Another lesson that stuck with me was a deep sense of gratitude for any energy and health I had to make it through each day.

CHOOSING A RECOVERY MINDSET
STUMBLING BLOCK OR SPRINGBOARD?

Recovery from cancer treatment is hard work. It doesn't happen overnight. We don't wake up from surgery completely healed. The initial physical recovery progresses into a more holistic recovery process. There may be setbacks and challenges along the way. I have found peace in a few new mindsets as I have walked through this last year of recovery.

I like to think of recovery as a process. It is something that I participate in every day with my actions, thoughts, and feelings. I have a choice in how I look at this difficult journey with breast cancer.

I could view cancer as a stumbling block and blame it for the troubles in my life. That would be a completely reasonable response. Cancer is difficult, and treatment is hard. It really had a negative impact on my marriage and made the months with my children difficult.

If I choose this mindset, I am welcoming bitterness and anger into my soul. As I examine this possibility along with my spiritual beliefs, I see that it doesn't fit. I have learned the most through some of the difficult times in my life. When the days are dark and full of fear, I turn to my faith for guidance and encouragement. I look through my journal entries on the most challenging days, and I see the record of how my faith brought me through it. I wrote out psalms of encouragement when I was facing the most frightening moments of my life. My family and friends were there for me in ways I couldn't have imagined. As I walked my recovery, did I want this cancer to be a source of bitterness and anger?

I needed a different vision. Ultimately, I decided that I would envision this particular time as a springboard for the next half of my life.

For years, I had been living with the fear of what others thought of me. I wanted to explore what my life might look like after raising my boys, but I was afraid of stepping out of my comfortable homemaker bubble. Cancer pushed me right out of that bubble. I never would have asked for this challenge, but it was my path. It was up to me to decide what was next.

CONCLUSION

MY DIAGNOSIS WITH DCIS in fall 2019 was a wake-up call. I had been drifting through my middle age, passing time while my kids grew up. I never spent much time thinking about my mortality; I just assumed that I had many more healthy years ahead of me.

In many ways, I was going through the motions. I was doing all the things I thought I should, and even beginning to explore some new educational avenues with my weekly French classes. But I wasn't feeling a sense of purpose and joy in my daily routines. I began to question if I was enjoying the last few years of my kids being at home, or if I was so exhausted that I looked forward to the break would come when they left home.

It was Halloween a few days after my surgery. My eldest son, Ken, had spent weeks preparing a concert for the trick-or-treaters who would come to our door. He had several seasonal songs ready to play that would guide kids to our home. Ken had spent hours each day practicing the music. On Halloween, he opened up our door and began playing the concert.

I am usually the one to open the door and greet the kids in their costumes. It is one of my favorite things to do, but I wasn't well enough to do that. Instead, I sat on the couch, curled up on a blanket, and just listened. There was nothing I would rather have done than listen to him play his music. I saw his body move to the music and enjoyed the expressiveness he brought to each song.

I remember thinking, "When was the last time that I just sat and listened to my son play?" Usually, I'm busy doing chores, cleaning up, or doing something else that would be more productive than listening to his music. In that moment, there was nothing I would rather be doing. I felt a deep sense of connection with him as I listened. I was physically, mentally, and emotionally present in a way that I hadn't been in years.

I cherish the memory of Halloween 2019. I was physically recovering from surgery, but emotionally present with my son in a way I hadn't been in years. As I continued in my treatment and recovery, I brought that moment with me. I wanted more of that in my life.

Over the last few years, I have made more of an effort to connect with and enjoy my sons. We have played video games, done puzzles, watched movies, and laughed together in a way that we hadn't done in years. Some of that was due to the forced togetherness of the pandemic, but most of it grew from the realization that our relationships would change soon. They would become adults and begin their own lives. I had a brief window of time before this change would happen. What type of connection did I want with them as adults?

Ken and Dan are young men now. They both tower over me and have deep, male voices. They are strong and capable. While I was undergoing treatment, they took on many of my daily responsibilities to help keep the household running and kept up with a challenging workload at school.

Dave has been working from home more than ever. I had thought our 20-year anniversary trip to France would be where we reconnected after my breast cancer. Instead, we have gone on long walks, snuggled together in our master retreat, and found ways to be romantic even with the teenagers just down the hall.

Throughout these past few years, I have worked to be present and enjoy my well-being after treatment. It hasn't been easy. We, like so many others, have had our lives radically changed.

My recovery year didn't look the way I thought it would, but I'm grateful for this unique way of closing out our family of four. Ken graduated in June 2021 and moved away to college. Dan is serving as ASB president for his virtual high school. As this book comes to publication, he will be preparing for graduation. My husband has had his work responsibilities expanded and now covers a much larger territory. Initially, I was concerned about the increase in business travel, but the coronavirus changed all of that. We had many more family dinners because we were all home together. The conversations have been rich, and laughter fills our home, especially when Dave decides to share his latest dad joke with us.

Sometime between Thanksgiving and Christmas 2020, I began to realize that I was feeling whole again. My physical health was the first to recover, but the mental and emotional toll of treatment took longer. I remember walking on the trails and watching the leaves drift off the trees. The previous fall, I had been in the middle of cancer treatment, and I was unsure what my future looked like. But this year, I felt a peace and a joy as I recognized that I had made it through this round of cancer.

I remember how scared I was at the beginning of my treatment. I heard the words of the doctors that this was treatable, but I didn't have any framework for believing them. I had never expected to have a breast cancer diagnosis at 41.

We cannot ever prepare for a diagnosis like this. It stops our lives and disrupts our work, family, and finances. I remember reading stories of women who walked through it before me, and I couldn't believe what they had been through. I had no idea how I was going to make it. I had plenty of support with my family and friends.

I encourage you to find ways to be kind and nurturing to yourself as you deal with these fears. Cancer is frightening. In 2021, my husband was treated for skin cancer on his nose. I watched him walk through the physical discomfort of the surgery and reconstruction, and the emotional aftermath of his changed appearance. There was nothing I could do to put the pieces back together for him except to be present. Watching him struggle with the recovery and question the validity of his emotions brought me right back to where I was at the beginning of my own treatment.

I never would have thought that breast cancer would be the diagnosis that helped me step out of my comfortable box at home and begin to write and connect with a larger audience. For that, I am grateful.

I have heard it said that cancer is the club that you never wanted to join, but it is filled with the most amazing people you will ever meet. As I have been researching, writing, and networking, I have connected with people all over the world. Breast cancer connects us. We share stories of diagnosis, treatments, side effects, fears, and also hope.

It is my hope for you that you find ways each day to prioritize your physical, mental, and emotional well-being during and after treatment so that you can cherish and enjoy the days ahead.

EPILOGUE

THE JOURNEY CONTINUES

a summer of uncertainty & another surgery

I WALKED INTO THE imaging office feeling anxious and unsettled. It had been almost three years since my first abnormal mammogram in 2019. The mammograms and ultrasounds had been normal since then. That was all about to change.

In June 2022, imaging on my left breast (the non-cancer side) revealed a mass that had grown significantly in six months. This finding was thought to be a benign fibroadenoma, and it had been changing in size slightly since it was notated on my chart in 2019. After several mammograms and an extensive set of ultrasounds, the radiologist decided to order a biopsy. As she described the procedure and next steps, my heart beat with terror. I knew exactly what was next and I wasn't looking forward to it.

My hands shook as I drove home. Was this cancer round two? I got home, collapsed into Dave's warm embrace, and let the emotions flow. Once I'd collected myself, I sent a message to my surgeon asking if he agreed with the referral for a biopsy. I hoped that he would spare me the procedure.

It was a Friday, so I spent the weekend worrying about my next steps. Note to self: Don't schedule imaging late on a Friday night. It makes for a worrisome weekend. My surgeon called me early the following the week and confirmed that a biopsy was needed. Okay, time to read my biopsy preparation tips and take my own advice.

I scheduled the biopsy for after our family vacation to New York. I didn't want to be dealing with recovery or results while we were sightseeing. It was a remarkable trip, but the worries were right under the surface, bubbling and brewing. I wasn't outwardly anxious, but my stomach distress throughout the trip told a different story.

At the beginning of July 2022, I had an ultrasound-guided biopsy on the lesion. It went smoothly, and I was surprised at how quickly I recovered. I took it easy for a few days and tried to distract myself until the results appointment. I had scheduled my appointment for six days after the biopsy, which I thought would be plenty of time for the pathology to come back.

I was mistaken. On Thursday, the day of my results appointment, I spent the entire day in an anxious spiral because the pathology wasn't back. Finally, at 5 p.m., the phone rang. It was my surgeon. "Hi Jennifer, how are you?"

"I don't know, you tell me." I quipped back at him. I was grateful for the call because I was tired of waiting for the pathology results. I didn't know just how much more uncertainty I could take.

"Your results are back, and the pathology board has reviewed them. There are spindle cells in the sample and results are inconclusive. They are recommending a lumpectomy. Let's get you in Tuesday for a pre-op."

Full stop. I had no idea biopsies could be inconclusive. I was facing another surgery. My heart sank as I thanked him profusely for the call, hung up, and sat down on the window seat. It was one thing to need a biopsy for a suspicious lesion, but now I was facing another lumpectomy for something inconclusive.

Just a few hours earlier I had been dancing in my kitchen because I'd signed a publication contract for this book. Now I was feeling overwhelmed and hopeless. What were spindle cells? I dove into research mode and quickly stopped. They could be benign or malignant and no amount of research would give me answers I longed for. Surgery was the only way out of this in-between.

Thankfully, I didn't have too much time to wait. Unlike my previous diagnosis process that had multiple rounds of imaging, biopsies, and genetic testing, this one was straightforward. Two weeks after the results call with my surgeon, I was headed to the hospital for another lumpectomy.

My lumpectomy in 2022 was a very different experience than the one I'd had in 2019. I was able to go to my local hospital, which was a short distance from my home. The last time I'd walked the halls as a patient was seventeen years earlier, in the labor and delivery department. Because of coronavirus protocols, Dave had to drop me off at the door of the hospital after my localization procedure was finished. I was grateful for the nurse navigators who were with me during the transition from localizing to the surgery department.

As I walked through this most recent surgery day, I felt peace and calm surround me every step of the way. The flow of this hospital made for a relaxing patient experience. Hospital check-in was done at the women's center right before localization, and so I was able to transition seamlessly from localizing to surgery. As I headed home after my lumpectomy, I hoped that this peaceful feeling would follow me.

My head spun in anxiety that first night after surgery. Now that the mass was out, the pathologists could test it. What would they find? Was I headed for more treatment? Would I need chemo or radiation? As Dave slept peacefully in bed next to me, I couldn't stop the internal panic. Finally, after doing some 2 a.m. research, I realized that the anxiety and insomnia was a side effect from the prescription pain medication I took right before bed. That was the one and only night I took that medicine!

A week after my lumpectomy, it was time for my first post-op appointment with my surgeon. Finally, it was time to get the pathology report. He read my chart and gave me the good news: it was benign. Then I saw a puzzled look cross his face. He realized that the report wasn't the final report from the hospital pathology department. He quickly apologized to me, and then got on the phone with the pathologist. "She's here in the room with me, when will that report be ready? Five minutes, fifteen minutes, an hour?"

He hung up and said that they wanted to have the head of breast pathology look at the final report to make a determination, but that it would be ready in about forty-five minutes. "Can I stay until it is ready?" I asked. I was done with the in-between of this summer. Did I have cancer again, or not?

"Sure. Just head out to the waiting room when we're done and I'll let you know when it's ready." After he checked my incisions and unwrapped me, I headed out to the waiting room to sit with Dave and wait.

After what felt like an eternity, he popped out from the back and gave me the good news. It was a benign fibroadenoma! There wasn't any more treatment needed. I felt all the tension release from my face. This latest scare was over.

As I progressed through this latest summer of in-between, it was a chance for me to reflect on the decisions that I made in 2019. If I had decided to have a mastectomy, I wouldn't have had this latest experience. Maybe if I had stayed on tamoxifen, the finding wouldn't have grown. There were a lot of things I could second-guess if I wanted to.

After much reflection, I decided that those trains of thought weren't helpful. I know exactly why I chose to have a lumpectomy in 2019. Those reasons are the same now as they were then. I was confident then in my decision, and that confidence enables me to deal with these new in-betweens as they come. My journey continues, and I proceed, one step at a time.

ACKNOWLEDGMENTS

THANK YOU TO MY husband, Dave. You never ceased to support me, whether that was holding me in my pain, or infusing a bit of well-timed humor into my treatment. You took over my jobs at home so I could recover, and you never stopped hoping for a joyful future together. Your encouragement during this writing process has kept me going, even when I felt like giving up.

Thank you to my sons, Ken and Dan, for persevering through these challenging times. You brought me heating pads and cold water, learned how to work with your dad during school, and became young men of depth and character. Thank you for putting up with all the dinner conversations that revolved around breasts!

To my mom, Linda. Thank you for finding all the laundry, coming to my appointments, and pulling so many weeds! Thank you for always encouraging me to follow my dreams, whether that was in dance, music, or writing.

To my dad, Greg, thank you for your words of experience and wisdom. You listened as my diagnosis twisted and turned, and you offered encouragement along the way. Thank you for your unending and steady love.

Rebekah, thank you for coming to my appointments, pulling me together after I received the news that I had breast cancer, and for your steady friendship for nearly two decades. You encourage me when I'm doubting my next steps and always have time to listen.

It has been said that it takes a village to get through cancer, and our situation was no different. Robin and Karen, my parents not by birth but by marriage, your love crossed state lines. I felt your prayers and encouragements throughout my cancer journey. Scott and Judee, thank you for being ready to help out whenever we asked. Knowing the boys had a place to go during surgery made it just a little easier to leave. Vaughn and Ronda, you were there to pray, surround us with support, and organize help for us. Thank you for your friendship. Bree, you were a consistent source of encouragement during my treatment and while I've been writing this book. I appreciate the spontaneous gifts and cheerful text messages.

We couldn't have walked through this time without the additional support of our extended family, friends, neighbors, and church family. Thank you for your prayers, words of encouragement, meals, flowers, and coffee deliveries!

To my medical team, a heartfelt thank you. To my surgeon, who always pursued the details and never stopped seeking the answers we needed, thank you. You walked me through a terrifying time with the confidence that comes with experience and dedication. To my oncologist, who took an appointment with me even before I had a diagnosis, thank you. No matter how busy your day was, I never felt rushed when I was in the room with you. To my radiation oncologist, thank you for patiently answering all my pre-treatment questions. I was nervous about transitioning to another medical group, and your calm demeanor and preparation eased my nerves. To my expanded medical team, radiologists, pathologists, techs, nurses, and office staff, a deep thank you. I had no idea how many people would be involved in my diagnosis and treatment, I'm grateful for the time you took with me to see me as a person and not simply a patient.

When I began writing this book, it was a very private affair. It felt like I was baring my soul when I reached out to find an editor. I've been fortunate to have had three who have shaped and formed this book into the one you hold in your hands today.

Claire Winters, you read the first draft, my outpouring of emotion, and saw not only what it was but what it could be. Thank you for seeing the potential and then teaching me how to construct a book that might benefit a reader rather than simply the author.

Bonnie Hearn Hill, you inspired me to think bigger. After reading and editing a few chapters, you implored me to send out query letters. You spent hours on the phone with me strategizing and encouraging me to keep querying.

To Nedah Rose, my editor at Bold Story Press, thank you. You patiently changed my whichs to thats, and back again! You refined the manuscript, encouraged me to persist through the many details that go into a finished book, and always brightened my day with your email close of "cheers."

To the incredible team at Bold Story Press, my deepest gratitude. You demonstrated care for me first as a woman and then as an author. The day I signed the book contract with you, I found out I needed surgery. My health and recovery from my unexpected 2022 surgery came first, and that says much about who you are as a publishing company.

Emily Barrosse, thank you for your vision for this book. When I wanted to narrow down my audience, you questioned why we wouldn't want to reach more women impacted by breast cancer. You believed in me, pursued me, and never stopped encouraging me during this journey. Julianna Scott Fein, my production director, thank you for sharing your experiences on the topics of breast health and imaging with me while you kept this project moving towards completion. To my book designer, Karen Polaski, I knew from our very first meeting, when I "just happened" to include a few of your covers on my inspiration list, that you would be able to capture the themes inside and create a beautiful book for my readers.

This book contains the words and experiences of many who have been impacted by cancer. Thank you for trusting me with your stories and encouraging me throughout this project. Thank you, Janna, Noelle, Jennifer F., Davita, Sandy, Jill, Lillian, Sue, Betty, Sheena, Nancy, Joni, Nanci, Melanie, Janelle, She, Mia, Amy, Flori, Jody, Claire, Dale, Cynthia, Lisa, Grace, and Dawn. Thank you to my beta readers, Jennifer W., Dr. Zavaleta, and Nancy. Thank you to the women in the California Breast Cancer Support group. I have learned much from our conversations online and in person.

In 2020, I began writing on my website and joined a vibrant worldwide cancer community. I have been encouraged, challenged, supported, and inspired by so many. Thank you to the #bcsm and medical community on Twitter. I appreciate the timely updates on research and new treatments. Thank you for amplifying my voice along with yours. I have grieved the deaths of many who died from cancer during my short time in the community. I dream of a day when treating breast cancer once is enough.

I've been asked, "When did you decide to become a writer?" and I often look back to my seventh grade English class with Ms. Friest. In her class, we spent one period writing and one period reading every day. It was there that I realized that I could pour my emotions out on the page and process them. Writing became a powerful and safe way to express myself. A few years later, Mrs. Raddatz challenged me to go beyond a first draft and use writing to inspire change in myself and others. For years, I dreamed of writing a book, but I never thought breast cancer would be the catalyst. I hope that by sharing my journey, you can find encouragement to take yours one step at a time.

APPENDIX

RESOURCES

THIS IS A LIVING list which will be updated as I discover more resources. To find the most current version of this appendix, including up-to-date links, please visit my website at https://jenniferadouglas.com. You can also connect with me on social media @mmejendouglas.

BOOKS

BREAST CANCER BOOKS–MEDICAL

Breast Cancer: Real Questions, Real Answers, David Chan, M.D.
The Breast Cancer Survival Manual, John Link M.D.
Dr. Susan Love's Breast Book, Susan Love, M.D.

BREAST CANCER BOOKS–MEMOIRS

Bald is Better with Earrings: A Survivor's Guide to Getting Through Breast Cancer, Andrea Hutton
Better: How I Let Go of Control, Held On to Hope, and Found Joy in My Darkest Hour, Amy Robach

CHEMOTHERAPY

Braving Chemo: What to Expect, How to Prepare and How to Get Through It, Beverly Zavaleta, M.D.

Getting Past the Fear: A Guide to Help You Mentally Prepare for Chemotherapy, Nancy Stordahl

OTHER BOOKS

The Big Ordeal: Coping with Cancer Emotions, Cynthia Hayes
Boundaries: When to Say Yes, How to Say No to Take Control of Your Life, Dr. Henry Cloud and Dr. John Townsend
Set Boundaries, Find Peace: A Guide to Reclaiming Yourself, Nedra Glover Tawwab

WEBSITES & FOUNDATIONS

American Cancer Society: https://cancer.org
- Resources for patients and caregivers
- Information for seeking support in all areas, including financial assistance

Breast Cancer.org: https://breastcancer.org
- Reliable information about treatments and understanding results
- Online support forums

Breast Cancer Research Foundation: https://www.bcrf.org
- Provides funding to breast cancer researchers
- Blog to share research news and resources

Dr. Susan Love Foundation: https://drsusanloveresearch.org
- Focuses on research to find the cause of breast cancer
- Educates through informative articles and videos

National Cancer Institute: https://cancer.gov
- Reliable and up-to-date information on treatments
- Information on survivorship
- Resources for caregivers and children

ASSEMBLING YOUR TEAM & TRAVEL

Who might be a part of your team: https://www.cancer.net/navigating-cancer-care/cancer-basics/cancer-care-team/oncology-team

Second Opinions: https://www.breastcancer.org/treatment/second_opinion/where

Travel

- City of Hope- International: https://www.cityofhope.org/patients/departments-and-services/center-for-international-medicine/patient-services/traveling-to-city-of-hope-international-patients
- City of Hope - Domestic Travel, https://www.cityofhope.org/patients/for-patients-and-visitors/accommodations-local-services-and-attractions
- Joe's House: Nonprofit that helps cancer patients find lodging options at a discount, https://www.joeshouse.org
- Johns Hopkins Medical Concierge Service: https://www.hopkinsmedicine.org/jhusa/patient_information/index.html

CAREGIVER SUPPORT

American Cancer Society Caregiver Resource Guide: https://www.cancer.org/treatment/caregivers/caregiver-resource-guide.html

Cancer Support Community/Gilda's Club: https://www.cancersupportcommunity.org

NCI Support for Caregivers of Cancer Patients: https://www.cancer.gov/about-cancer/coping/caregiver-support

FINANCIAL RESOURCES

CancerCare-Resources for the East Coast of the USA, https://www.cancercare.org

CDC: https://www.cdc.gov/cancer/survivors/patients/paying-for-cancer-treatment.htm

- Good list of resources with ideas to help pay for care

Living Beyond Breast Cancer Fund: https://www.lbbc.org/about-us/what-we-do/lbbc-fund

FINDING CANCER CARE

American Society for Breast Surgeons: https://www.breastsurgeons.org

- Breast 360: https://breast360.org

American Society for Clinical Oncologists—choosing a cancer treatment center

- https://www.cancer.net/navigating-cancer-care/managing-your-care/choosing-cancer-treatment-center

Comprehensive cancer centers: National Comprehensive Cancer Network

- https://www.nccn.org/home
- https://www.nccn.org/patientresources/patient-resources/guidelines-for-patients
- NCI designated cancer center, https://www.cancer.gov/research/infrastructure/cancer-centers

HOUSECLEANING

Cleaning for a Reason: https://cleaningforareason.org

https://castle-keepers.com/how-do-you-clean-for-a-cancer-patient/

INTERNATIONAL CANCER RESOURCES

Breast Cancer Now, UK: https://breastcancernow.org
Breast Cancer Society of Canada: https://bcsc.ca/about-us/
Canadian Breast Cancer Network: https://www.cbcn.ca/en/
Cancer Research UK: https://www.cancerresearchuk.org/about-cancer/breast-cancer
UK National Health Services: https://www.nhs.uk/conditions/breast-cancer/

METASTATIC BREAST CANCER RESOURCES

Advanced Breast Cancer: Educational and support resources for people living with advanced and metastatic breast cancer. https://advancedbreastcancer.net
Living Beyond Breast Cancer- Living with Metastatic Breast Cancer: https://www.lbbc.org/your-journey/living-with-metastatic-breast-cancer
Metavivor: Research and support for those living with metastatic breast cancer. https://www.metavivor.org
Project Life: A membership-based virtual wellness house for those living with metastatic breast cancer and their loved ones. http://www.projectlifembc.com
Twisted Pink: Advocacy and education for people living with metastatic breast cancer. https://www.twistedpink.org

USEFUL ITEMS DURING TREATMENT & RECOVERY

Anaono Intimates: Specially designed bras and loungewear for breast cancer patients

Fruit of the Loom Front Close Sports Bra
Drain pouch
Shirts with drain pockets
Recovery robe (Brobe)
Skincare during radiation

- Aquaphor
- Avene thermal water
- Avene Xeracalm A.D
- Calendula
- Udderly Smooth

ADDITIONAL RESOURCES & BLOGS

Agendia Genomic Tests: Offers two precision genomic tests to help oncologists plan care. Their tests assess recurrence risk and also test the biomarkers of tumor samples. https://agendia.com/our-tests/

Breast Cancer Freebies: Collection of free resources available for breast cancer patients and their families. Includes list of retreats. https://breastcancerfreebies.com

Caring Bridge: A website designed to support people going on health journeys. Offers a way to share health updates with customized privacy settings. https://caringbridge.org.

DiepC Journey and Foundation: Provides education and information about breast reconstruction options after mastectomy. https://diepcjourney.com

DCISionRT: Genomic test to help assess the potential benefit of radiation treatment for DCIS patients. https://preludedx.com/dcisionrt/

His Breast Cancer Awareness: Information and support for men with breast cancer. https://www.hisbreastcancer.org/about-his.

Journeying Beyond Breast Cancer: Blog with weekly roundup posts from around the cancer community. https://journeyingbeyondbreastcancer.com

Male Breast Cancer Global Alliance: Advocacy, community, and research for men with breast cancer. https://mbcglobalalliance.org/.

Male Breast Cancer Patient Guide: Information about male breast cancer and treatment. https://www.cancer.gov/types/breast/patient/male-breast-treatment-pdq.

MOLLI Surgical H.O.P.E. Project: A collection of resources, interviews, support, and services assembled by breast cancer clinicians and advocates put together and maintained by MOLLI Surgical. You might even find me on their wall! http://mollisurgical.com/hope/

Nancy's Point: Breast Cancer blog with many informative resources and books about her cancer diagnosis and treatment, making surgical decisions, and facing chemotherapy. https://nancyspoint.com

No Half Measures: Metastatic breast cancer blog by Abigail Johnston. https://nohalfmeasures.blog

Oncotype Testing: Exact Sciences does genomic testing on pathology samples to help determine the potential benefit of chemotherapy. Also has testing for DCIS. https://precisiononcology.exactsciences.com/healthcare-providers/treatment-determination/breast-cancer

Surviving Breast Cancer: Free events and resources for breast cancer patients and their families. https://www.survivingbreastcancer.org

Understanding a Breast Pathology Report on Youtube: Series of informative videos about reading and interpreting pathology reports. https://www.youtube.com/channel/UC6VYKQlVo8DS5TzuvS8C_FA/featured

ENDNOTES

1 First Emotion I'm Overwhelmed

1 Jennifer, email correspondence to author, November 5, 2020.
2 Noelle, email correspondence to author, November 8, 2020.
3 Davita, email correspondence to author, January 21, 2021.

2 Choosing a Surgeon & Getting a Second Opinion

1 "Cancer Centers," National Cancer Institute, 2022, https://cancercenters.cancer.gov/Center/CancerCenters.
2 *NCI Dictionary of Cancer Terms*, National Cancer Institute, 2022, https://www.cancer.gov/publications/dictionaries/cancer-terms.
3 "Specialty of General Surgery," the American Board of Surgery, February 2017, https://www.absurgery.org/default.jsp?aboutsurgerydefined.
4 "Financial Toxicity (Financial Distress) and Cancer Treatment (PDQ®)–Patient Version," National Cancer Institute, 2019, https://www.cancer.gov/about-cancer/managing-care/track-care-costs/financial-toxicity-pdq.
5 Konish, Lorie, "This is the real reason most Americans file for bankruptcy," CNBC (website), February 11, 2019, https://www.cnbc.com/2019/02/11/this-is-the-real-reason-most-americans-file-for-bankruptcy.html.
6 Sandy, personal correspondence to author via Facebook Messenger, June 8, 2021.

7 Noelle, email, 2020.
8 Jill, email correspondence to author, November 4, 2020.
9 Lillian, email correspondence to author, November 3, 2020.
10 Davita, email, 2021.

3 **Imaging** Learning a New Language (Besides French) in My Forties

1 "Calcification," *NCI Dictionary of Cancer Terms*, National Cancer Institute, 2021, https://www.cancer.gov/publications/dictionaries/cancer-terms/def/calcification.
2 Bjørn Helge Østerås, Anne Catrine T. Martinsen, Randi Gullien, and Per Skaane, "Digital Mammography versus Breast Tomosynthesis: Impact of Breast Density on Diagnostic Performance in Population-based Screening," *Radiology*, August 13, 2019, https://doi.org/10.1148/radiol.2019190425.
3 "Mammograms," National Cancer Institute, December 7, 2016, https://www.cancer.gov/types/breast/mammograms-fact-sheet#how-are-screening-and-diagnostic-mammograms-different.
4 "Do I Need a Breast MRI," Breast360.org (website by The American Society of Breast Surgeons Foundation), 2017, https://breast360.org/topic/2017/01/01/do-i-need-breast-mri/.
5 Bernadette M. Greenwood, "Breast MRI: All About Timing," *Imaging Technology News*, September 17, 2009, https://www.itnonline.com/article/breast-mri-all-about-timing.
6 "What Is an MRI With Contrast?" Envision Radiology, https://www.envrad.com/what-is-an-mri-with-contrast/.
7 "Mammograms," National Cancer Institute, https://www.cancer.gov/types/breast/mammograms-fact-sheet.
8 "Mammograms—What Is the Breast Imaging Reporting and Database System (BI-RADS)?" National Cancer Institute, December 7, 2016, https://www.cancer.gov/types/breast/mammograms-fact-sheet#what-is-the-breast-imaging-reporting-and-database-system-BI-RADS.

9 "Dense Breasts: Answers to Commonly Asked Questions," National Cancer Institute, July 14, 2020, https://www.cancer.gov/types/breast/breast-changes/dense-breasts.
10 Noelle, email, 2020.
11 Jill, email, 2021.
12 Lillian, email, 2020

4 **Biopsies, So Many Biopsies** Is This Over Yet?

1 "Vasogagal Syncope," Mayo Clinic (website), https://www.mayoclinic.org/diseases-conditions/vasovagal-syncope/symptoms-causes/syc-20350527.
2 Fred Burbank, M.D., "Stereotactic Breast Biopsy: Its History, Its Present, and Its Future." *The American Surgeon* 62, no.2 (1996): 128–50.
3 *"Liquid Biopsy: Using DNA in Blood to Detect, Track, and Treat Cancer,"* National Cancer Institute, November 8, 2017, https://www.cancer.gov/news-events/cancer-currents-blog/2017/liquid-biopsy-detects-treats-cancer.
4 Dr. Mohammad Taghi Niknejad, "Breast imaging-reporting and data system (BI-RADS)," *Radiopaedia*, August 21, 2022, https://doi.org/10.53347/rID-10003.
5 "Breast biopsy," Mayo Clinic (website), https://www.mayoclinic.org/tests-procedures/breast-biopsy/about/pac-20384812.
6 Davita, email, 2021.
7 Noelle, email, 2020.
8 Sue, personal correspondence to author via Facebook Messenger, September 27, 2022.
9 "U.S. Federal Rule Mandates Open Notes," OpenNotes.org, September 15, 2022, https://www.opennotes.org/onc-federal-rule/.
10 Dr. Caragh Behan, "The benefits of meditation and mindfulness practices during times of crisis such as COVID-19," *Irish Journal of Psychological Medicine*, 37, no. 4 (2020): 256–258, https://doi.org/10.1017/ipm.2020.38.

5 **Diagnosis Day** Really? Breast Cancer for My Birthday?

1 "Understanding my Report," Johns Hopkins University, https://pathology.jhu.edu/breast/understand-report/.
2 "Breast Changes and Conditions," National Cancer Institute, June 29, 2019, https://www.cancer.gov/types/breast/breast-changes#breast-changes-that-are-not-cancer.
3 "Extensive Lymph Node Removal Doesn't Improve Survival in Some Women with Early-Stage Breast Cancer," National Cancer Institute, October 10, 2017, https://www.cancer.gov/news-events/cancer-currents-blog/2017/breast-cancer-lymph-node-removal.
4 Karthik Giridhar, M.D., "HER2-positive breast cancer: What is it?" Mayo Clinic, April 7, 2020, https://www.mayoclinic.org/breast-cancer/expert-answers/faq-20058066.
5 Molly Adams, "HER2 low breast cancer expert: Precise diagnosis can lead to personalized treatment," University of Texas M.D. Anderson Center, September 9, 2022, https://www.mdanderson.org/cancerwise/her2-low-breast-cancer-expert--precise-diagnosis-can-lead-to-personalized-treatment.h00-159542901.html.
6 Greg, personal correspondence to author, October 29, 2020.
7 Linda, personal correspondence to author, 2020.
8 Davita, email, 2021.
9 Jennifer, email, 2020.
10 Jill, email, 2020.
11 Betty, personal correspondence via Facebook Messenger, October 10, 2022.
12 "NCI Dictionary of Cancer Terms," National Institutes of Health, https://www.cancer.gov/publications/dictionaries/cancer-terms.
13 "Cancer And Mental Health," Mental Health America, https://www.mhanational.org/cancer-and-mental-health.

6 **Making a Surgical Game Plan**

1 "Women's Health and Cancer Rights Act (WHCRA)," U.S. Department of Labor, https://www.dol.gov/agencies/ebsa/laws-and-regulations/laws/whcra.

2 E. Shelley Hwang, Terry Hyslop et al., "The COMET (Comparison of Operative versus Monitoring and Endocrine Therapy) trial: a phase III randomised controlled clinical trial for low-risk ductal carcinoma in situ (DCIS)" *BMJ Open*, 2019, vol 9, issue 3, https://bmjopen.bmj.com/content/9/3/e026797.

3 "Breast Reconstruction After Mastectomy," National Cancer Institute, February 24, 2017, https://www.cancer.gov/types/breast/reconstruction-fact-sheet.

4 "Aesthetic Flat Closure," *NCI Dictionary of Cancer Terms*, National Cancer Institute, https://www.cancer.gov/publications/dictionaries/cancer-terms/def/aesthetic-flat-closure.

5 Heather Richardson and Grace Ma, "The Goldilocks mastectomy," *International Journal of Surgery*, 10, No. 9 (2012): 522–526, https://doi.org/10.1016/j.ijsu.2012.08.003.

6 Dr. Anne Peled, "Breast and Nipple Sensation Preserving Mastectomy," https://annepeledmd.com/2020/03/breast-and-nipple-sensation-preserving-mastectomy/.

7 Bernard Fisher, M.D., Stewart Anderson, Ph.D., "Twenty-Year Follow-up of a Randomized Trial Comparing Total Mastectomy Lumpectomy, and Lumpectomy plus Irradiation for the Treatment of Invasive Breast Cancer," *New England Journal of Medicine*, 347, no. 16 (2002): 1233–41, https://doi.org/10.1056/NEJMoa022152.

8 American Society for Breast Surgeons, "Consensus Guidelines on Breast Cancer Lumpectomy Margins," December 20, 2017, https://www.breastsurgeons.org/docs/statements/Consensus-Guideline-on-Breast-Cancer-Lumpectomy-Margins.pdf.

9 Jeffrey Landercasper, Eric Whitacre et al., "Reasons for re-excision after lumpectomy for breast cancer: insight from the American Society of Breast Surgeons Mastery (SM) database," *Annals of Surgical Oncology*, 21, no. 10 (2014): 3185–91, https://pubmed.ncbi.nlm.nih.gov/25047472/.

10 SeungSang Ko, Yi Kyeong Chun et al., "The Usefulness of Intraoperative Circumferential Frozen-Section Analysis of Lumpectomy Margins in Breast-Conserving Surgery," *Journal of Breast Cancer*, 20, no. 2 (2017):176–182, https://pubmed.ncbi.nlm.nih.gov/28690654/.

11 Narendra Nath Basu, James Hodson et al., "The Angelina Jolie effect: Contralateral risk-reducing mastectomy trends in patients at increased risk of breast cancer," *Scientific Reports*, 11, no. 1 (2021): 2847. Published online February 2, 2021, https://doi.org/10.1038/s41598-021-82654-x.

12 "Breast and Ovarian Cancer and Family History Risk Categories," Center for Disease Control, March 25, 2020, https://www.cdc.gov/genomics/disease/breast_ovarian_cancer/risk_categories.htm.

13 "BRCA Gene Mutations: Cancer Risk and Genetic Testing," National Cancer Institute, November 19, 2020, https://www.cancer.gov/about-cancer/causes-prevention/genetics/brca-fact-sheet.

14 "MolDX: BRCA1 and BRCA2 Testing," Medicare Coverage Database, February 16, 2017, https://www.cms.gov/medicare-coverage-database/details/lcd-details.aspx?LCDId=36813.

15 Jennifer, email, 2020.

16 Lillian, email, 2020.

17 Noelle, email, 2020.

18 Davita, email, 2021.

19 Sheena, email to author, September 27, 2022.

7 **Preparation for Surgery** So Many Things to Do

1 Anuj Shah, Corey J. Hayes et al., "Characteristics of Initial Prescription Episodes and Likelihood of Long-Term Opioid Use—United States, 2006–2015." *Morbidity and Mortality Weekly Report, CDC*, Rep, 17, no. 66 (2017): 265–269, http://dx.doi.org/10.15585/mmwr.mm6610a1.

2 Stephanie Lam, M.S., Helena Qu, B.S. et al., "Trends in Peripheral Nerve Block Usage in Mastectomy and Lumpectomy: Analysis of a National Database From 2010 to 2018," *Anesthesia & Analgesia*, 133, No. 1 (2021): 32–40, https://journals.lww.com/anesthesia-analgesia/Fulltext/2021/07000/Trends_in_Peripheral_Nerve_Block_Usage_in.7.aspx.
3 Noelle, email, 2020.
4 Nancy, personal correspondence to author via Facebook Messenger, September 30, 2022.
5 Joni, personal correspondence to author via Facebook Messenger, September 30, 2022.

8 **Surgery Day** Facing the Unknown

1 Megha Madhukar Kapoor, Miral Mahesh Patel, and Marion Elizabeth Scoggins, "The Wire and Beyond: Recent Advances in Breast Imaging Preoperative Needle Localization," *RadioGraphics*, 39, no. 7 (2019): 1886–1906, https://doi.org/10.1148/rg.2019190041.
2 Megan Kalambo, M.D., Basak E Dogan, M.D., Gary J Whitman, M.D.,"Step by Step: Planning a Needle Localization Procedure," *Clinical Imaging*, 60, no.1 (2020): 100–108, https://www.ncbi.nlm.nih.gov/pmc/articles/PMC8635082/.
3 Sandy, Facebook Messenger, 2021.
4 Noelle, email, 2020.
5 Janelle, email to author, October 6, 2022.

9 **Soft Landing** Optimizing for Early Recovery

1 Jill, email, 2020.
2 Davita, email, 2021.
3 Jennifer, email, 2020.

10 **The Beat Goes On** Oncology & Post-Surgical Choices

1 "Cancer Stat Facts: Female Breast Cancer Subtypes," National Cancer Institute, https://seer.cancer.gov/statfacts/html/breast-subtypes.html.

2 "Stages of Breast Cancer," National Institute of Cancer, https://www.cancer.gov/types/breast/patient/breast-treatment-pdq#_148.

3 Dr. Pragnya Chigurupati, "Understanding the Staging of Breast Cancer," August 24, 2021, https://drpragnya.com/blog/understanding-the-staging-of-breast-cancer/.

4 "Tumor Markers in Common Use," National Cancer Institute, https://www.cancer.gov/about-cancer/diagnosis-staging/diagnosis/tumor-markers-list.

5 "Treatment Option Overview," National Cancer Institute, https://www.cancer.gov/types/breast/patient/breast-treatment-pdq#_185.

6 "Radiation therapy for breast cancer," Mayo Clinic, https://www.mayoclinic.org/tests-procedures/radiation-therapy-for-breast-cancer/about/pac-20384940.

7 "Drugs Approved for Breast Cancer," National Cancer Institute, https://www.cancer.gov/about-cancer/treatment/drugs/breast.

8 "Tamoxifen Side Effects," Drugs.com, https://www.drugs.com/sfx/tamoxifen-side-effects.html.

9 Monica Morrow, "Refining the Use of Endocrine Therapy for Ductal Carcinoma in Situ," *Journal of Clinical Oncology*, 30, no. 12 (April 20, 2012): 1249–1251, March 4, 2012, https://ascopubs.org/doi/full/10.1200/JCO.2011.40.5514.

10 Noelle, email, 2020.

11 Davita, email, 2021.

12 Jill, email, 2020.

13 Jennifer, email, 2020.

14 Janelle, email, 2022.

11 **Radiation** Bring Headphones

1 Miriam A. Knoll, M.D., Daniel Aruch, M.D., "Contemporary Clinical Oncology Training in the United States: Is Radiation or Medical Oncology Right for You?" *ASCO Connection*, August 4, 2015, https://connection.asco.org/blogs/contemporary-clinical-oncology-training-united-states-radiation-or-medical-oncology-right-you.

2 Greg Kennelty, "Role of Radiation Continues to Change in Elderly Patients with Breast Cancer," *Cure Today*, June 1, 2016, https://www.curetoday.com/view/role-of-radiation-continues-to-change-in-elderly-patients-with-breast-cancer.

3 "Radiation Therapy to Treat Cancer," National Cancer Institute, https://www.cancer.gov/about-cancer/treatment/types/radiation-therapy.

4 Chao-Pin Hsiao, Barbara Daly, Leorey N. Saligan, "The Etiology and management of radiotherapy-induced fatigue," *Expert Review of Quality of Life in Cancer Care*, 1, no. 4 (2016): 323–328. https://doi.org/10.1080/23809000.2016.1191948.

5 Joni, Facebook Messenger, 2022.

6 Nancy, Facebook Messenger, 2022.

7 Nanci, personal correspondence to author via Facebook Messenger, September 27, 2022.

12 **Breast Cancer Swirl** Handling Complex Post-Treatment Emotions (Yours & Theirs)

1 "Cancer-Related Post-traumatic Stress (PDQ)-Patient Version," National Cancer Institute, July 9, 2019, https://www.cancer.gov/about-cancer/coping/survivorship/new-normal/ptsd-pdq.

2 Davita, email, 2021.

3 Noelle, email, 2020.

4 Jill, email, 2020.

5 Jennifer, email, 2020.

6 Patricia A. Ganz, M.D., and Kathleen Van Dyk, Ph.D., "Cognitive Impairments in Patients with Breast Cancer: Understanding the Impact of Chemotherapy and Endocrine Therapy," *Journal of Clinical Oncology*, 38, Issue 17, April 9, 2020, https://ascopubs.org/doi/10.1200/JCO.20.00336.

13 **Sex. Yes, Sex** (or Lack Thereof)

1 Mia Spano-Curtiss & Sondra Price, @BSbreastcancer, Twitter, September 29, 2022, https://twitter.com/bsbreastcancer/status/1575544759757598720?s=46&t=ZQ5NRe6KGkxmmXXLd8TpzQ.

2 Kate, @kati_hargreaves, Twitter, September 29, 2022. https://twitter.com/kati_hargreaves/status/1575572443636195328?s=61&t=cMbfgld3Atu3SH6EUmbqpg.

3 Flori, @CANsurvive, Twitter, September 29, 2022, https://twitter.com/cansurvive/status/1575520424863027200?s=21&t=SmouvOoNC7Lrfc2B34tmcA.

4 Jody Hinkle, @Jody_Hinkle, Twitter, September 29, 2022, https://twitter.com/jody_hinkle/status/1575556306332962816?s=46&t=ZQ5NRe6KGkxmmXXLd8TpzQ.

5 She, @ShehasMBC, Twitter, September 29, 2022, https://twitter.com/shehasmbc/status/1575594486612525056?s=46&t=Yl4M6kpPPJn_7Xk0os1ykQ.

14 **Finding a New Beautiful** Getting to Know the Post-Cancer You

1 "Lymphedema," Mayo Clinic, https://www.mayoclinic.org/diseases-conditions/lymphedema/diagnosis-treatment/drc-20374687.

2 Rowan T. Chlebowski, "Nutrition and physical activity influence on breast cancer incidence and outcome," *The Breast*, 22, Suppl 2 (August 2013): S30-7. doi: 10.1016/j.breast.2013.07.006. PMID: 24074789.

3 Dawn, Facebook Messenger, 2022.

4 Janelle, email, 2022.

5 Grace, personal correspondence to author via Facebook Messenger, October 6, 2022.

ABOUT THE AUTHOR

JENNIFER A. DOUGLAS IS a writer and breast cancer patient advocate. A routine annual mammogram in 2019 revealed her breast cancer at stage zero and upended her daily homemaking and virtual schooling routines. Instead of organizing the lessons for the day, she found herself researching the many treatment decisions before her. She quickly learned that a breast cancer diagnosis impacts the entire family.

After the end of treatment, she felt called to encourage other patients through her writing and social media presence. Her patient advocacy efforts focus on the challenges facing early-stage breast cancer patients during their diagnosis, treatment, and recovery.

Her advocacy and encouraging voice is a welcomed addition to the breast cancer community. She was named a 2022 Breast Cancer Awareness Month influencer by the Susan Love Foundation. In 2022, she was invited to be a part of the inaugural Amgen Oncology Educational Social Media Summit focusing on addressing the barrier to cancer care facing all cancer patients. She has hosted episodes of "Breast Practices," as a part of MOLLI Surgical's H.O.P.E.

program, which encourages breast cancer patients and their families during their journeys.

Jennifer's writing has been featured in HealthGrades as a part of their Treating Breast Cancer Early series in 2022, and also on Surviving Breast Cancer's blog.

In addition to partnering with foundations and industry, and writing regularly on her blog, Jennifer is also active encouraging breast cancer patients in her local community. She hosts a weekly video chat for the California Breast Cancer Facebook Group and meets in-person monthly with local breast cancer survivors.

When she isn't advocating and encouraging others in her Southern California breast cancer community, she enjoys reading, drinking coffee, speaking French, and walking with her husband and their beagles.

Jennifer can be found on her website, https://jenniferadouglas.com, and on social media, @mmejendouglas. *A Breast Cancer Journey: Living it One Step at a Time* is her debut book.

ABOUT BOLD STORY PRESS

BOLD STORY PRESS IS a curated, woman-owned hybrid publishing company with a mission of publishing well-written stories by women. If your book is chosen for publication, our team of expert editors and designers will work with you to publish a professionally edited and designed book. Every woman has a story to tell. If you have written yours and want to explore publishing with Bold Story Press, contact us at https://boldstorypress.com.

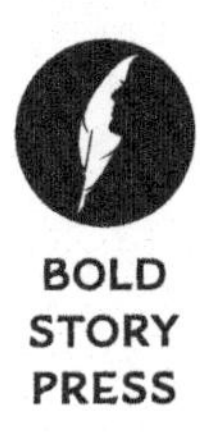

The Bold Story Press logo, designed by Grace Arsenault, was inspired by the nom de plume, or pen name, a sad necessity at one time for female authors who wanted to publish. The woman's face hidden in the quill is the profile of Virginia Woolf, who, in addition to being an early feminist writer, founded and ran her own publishing company, Hogarth Press.

Made in the USA
Monee, IL
23 May 2023